Words of Praise

'A valuable and informative guide for any woman experiencing
problems with fertility.'
Joan Z. Borysenko, Ph.D., the best-selling author of
Inner Peace for Busy Women

'At last! A simple, accurate, and empowering message for
the thousands of women diagnosed with PCOS.'
Christiane Northrup, MD.

PCOS

AND YOUR

FERTILITY

PCOS

AND YOUR
FERTILITY

Your Guide to Self-Care,
Emotional Wellbeing and
Medical Support

COLETTE HARRIS and THERESA CHEUNG

HAY HOUSE

Australia • Canada • Hong Kong • India
South Africa • United Kingdom • United States

First published and distributed in the United Kingdom by:
Hay House UK Ltd, 292B Kensal Rd, London W10 5BE. Tel.: (44) 20 8962 1230; Fax: (44) 20 8962 1239. www.hayhouse.co.uk

Published and distributed in the United States of America by:
Hay House, Inc., PO Box 5100, Carlsbad, CA 92018-5100. Tel.: (1) 760 431 7695 or (800) 654 5126; Fax: (1) 760 431 6948 or (800) 650 5115. www.hayhouse.com

Published and distributed in Australia by:
Hay House Australia Ltd, 18/36 Ralph St, Alexandria NSW 2015. Tel.: (61) 2 9669 4299; Fax: (61) 2 9669 4144. www.hayhouse.com.au

Published and distributed in the Republic of South Africa by:
Hay House SA (Pty), Ltd, PO Box 990, Witkoppen 2068. Tel./Fax: (27) 11 467 8904. www.hayhouse.co.za

Published and distributed in India by:
Hay House Publishers India, Muskaan Complex, Plot No.3, B-2, Vasant Kunj, New Delhi – 110 070. Tel.: (91) 11 4176 1620; Fax: (91) 11 4176 1630. www.hayhouse.co.in

Distributed in Canada by:
Raincoast, 9050 Shaughnessy St, Vancouver, BC V6P 6E5. Tel.: (1) 604 323 7100; Fax: (1) 604 323 2600

Copyright © 2004 by Colette Harris and Theresa Cheung.
Revised and updated © 2011.

The moral rights of the authors have been asserted.

The authors of this book does not dispense medical advice or prescribe the use of any technique as a form of treatment for physical or medical problems without the advice of a physician, either directly or indirectly. The intent of the authors is only to offer information of a general nature to help you in your quest for emotional and spiritual wellbeing. In the event you use any of the information in this book for yourself, which is your constitutional right, the authors and the publisher assume no responsibility for your actions.

A catalogue record for this book is available from the British Library.

ISBN 978-1-84850-491-2

Printed and bound in Great Britain by TJ International, Padstow, Cornwall

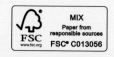

Dedication

For women with PCOS and the people who support them

Contents

Acknowledgements

Colette:

A big thank you to Theresa for being such a great, enthusiastic and energetic colleague; to Hay House for being so supportive and helpful; to Chris for his steadfast support and kindness; to everyone at Verity and in the international PCOS community for their hard work getting PCOS on the map; to all the women who have contacted me and Theresa to share their stories and thoughts on dealing with PCOS – we couldn't have done it without you.

Theresa:

Thank you to Colette for being such an inspiration and joy to work with. Thank you to our editor, Michelle Pilley, for her support and encouragement. Thank you to Hay House. Thank you to Ray, and to my two beautiful children, Robert and Ruth, for their patience and love while I completed this project. Thank you to the many women with PCOS I spoke to in the course of writing this book. I am truly grateful for the insight you gave me.

Colette and Theresa:

Thank you to all the experts and advisors listed below for giving their time and thought to the questions asked and sharing their knowledge with us and/or their important research on PCOS and fertility.

Dr Adam Balen – Consultant Obstetrician and Gynecologist and Subspecialist in reproductive medicine and surgery, Leeds General Infirmary

Frances Box – B.A., M.A.R., M.I.F.A., I.I.S.T., I.C.A.S., I.T.E.C., Raw. Dip. Reflexologist & Aromatherapist

Lucy Broughton – Health journalist

Umahro Cadogan – Lecturer at the Danish Institute of Optimal Nutrition

Bernice Chiswell – Bsc SRD. Senior Dietitian, Bedford Hospital, UK

Dr Gerard Conway – Consultant Gynaecologist, Middlesex Hospital, London

Dr Alice Domar – Harvard Medical School, Mind/Body research program

Dr James Douglas – Reproductive Endocrinologist, Plano Medical Center, Plano, Texas

Dr Robert Franklin – Clinical Professor of Obstetrics and Gynecology, Baylor College of Medicine, Houston, Texas.

Prof Stephen Franks – Professor of Reproductive Endocrinology, Imperial College, London

Jacqui Garnier MAR – Reflexologist, London

Dr Marilyn Glenville – Nutritional therapist

Prof Gabor Kovacs – Director of Obstetrics and Gynecology, Monash University, Melbourne, Australia

Dr Neils Lauersen – Obstetrician and Gynecologist, St Vincent Medical Center, New York

Dr Helen Mason – Senior Lecturer in Reproductive Endocrinology, St George's Hospital Medical School, London

Jules McClean – BA, Couns. Adv.Dip.Couns. M B A C P (Accred), counsellor and psychotherapist

Denise Tiran – MSc RM RGN ADM PGCEA, midwife, university lecturer, aromatherapist

Dr Samuel Thatcher – Expert in reproductive endocrinology serving on the Advisory Board of the American Infertility Association

Dr Ann Walker – Medical herbalist and nutrition research scientist,

Toni Weschler – Fertility Awareness Counselling and Training Seminars

Introduction

'I've just been diagnosed with PCOS and told it means I might not be able to have children! What on earth is this condition? And how can I make sure it doesn't affect me this way?' CHARLOTTE, 26

'I've got PCOS and the clock is ticking. I haven't met Mr. Right yet and sometimes wonder if I ever will. I want to have children and I'm seriously considering becoming a single mother by choice.' RACHEL, 35

'I don't want to have kids right now as I just don't feel ready, but I'm worried that PCOS will affect my future chances of getting pregnant when the time is right for me.' JENNY, 24

You may be reading this book because you have polycystic ovarian syndrome (PCOS) and have been trying for a baby, without success, for some time now. Problems with fertility are the number one reason why women visit their doctor and end up being diagnosed with PCOS. Perhaps you have PCOS and you are worried about how the condition may impact on your chances of motherhood in the future, or perhaps you are pregnant and worried about being a high-risk pregnancy.

If fertility is a concern for you, you're certainly not alone. Research shows that women with PCOS are more concerned about their fertility than women without, and that this can affect their quality of life.[1] The first question many women with PCOS ask, even if they don't want a baby right now, is: 'Will I be able to have babies when the time is right for me?'

If you have PCOS, fertility is a big issue. When your periods are irregular or absent and there are problems with ovulation, you're more likely to have problems. Without an egg in the right place at the right time to receive a sperm, you can't get pregnant. And even if all this happens, the incidence of miscarriage for women with PCOS is thought to be higher than average.[2] But don't panic. Here's the good news:

THE GOOD NEWS

Recent studies show that many women with PCOS get pregnant and give birth to healthy babies readily, once they get some key symptoms under control by balancing underlying hormone levels. And in many cases these pregnancies occur without fertility drugs.[3]

'Over 70 percent of women with PCOS do manage to conceive naturally in the end. Over 20 percent manage to conceive with treatment. There is much hope and considerable help for PCOS patients to establish a pregnancy,' says renowned expert in reproductive endocrinology, Dr Samuel Thatcher. 'Therapy may be as much as 90 percent effective for fertility problems related to PCOS.'

HOW THIS BOOK WORKS

This book is designed to help you maximize your chances of being able to get pregnant and have a healthy pregnancy. It provides a practical handbook for you to work through as you go on your fertility journey.

Chapters One and Two
Chapter One explains what PCOS is. Then, whatever stage of the journey you're currently at, the Seven-Step Fertility-Boosting action plan

in Chapter Two is a basic set of guidelines for women with PCOS to follow, to help maximize their ability to conceive. It will work as a primer for you even if you're not ready to start trying just yet; as a booster if you are trying; and as the foundation for a self-care plan that can be fine-tuned especially for you if you find you need some extra help.

Chapter Three

That's where Chapter Three comes in – if you've tried the seven steps and you're still dealing with niggling problems such as irregular periods, then use the scientifically-backed information in this section to fine-tune the basic plan by using a proactive approach to self care and natural therapies that you and your partner can embark on together.

Chapters Four and Five

If you want or need to consider natural or medical fertility treatment, Chapters Four and Five look at what's on offer to you as a woman with PCOS. These treatments will work in conjunction with the Seven-Step plan, which is still your basic self-help plan and will help enhance the effects of any treatment your undertake.

Chapter Six

Happily, as so many women with PCOS do eventually conceive, this chapter looks at how you can have a healthy pregnancy with PCOS.

Chapters Seven and Eight

All of this can be quite an exhausting process not only physically, but mentally too. So Chapters Seven and Eight are full of practical information to help you ride the ups and downs of the PCOS fertility rollercoaster, and stay happy and healthy while you're riding it.

PERSONAL PCOS STORIES

Because we know ourselves that sometimes the best medicine for helping you cope with PCOS is hearing the stories of other women who have the condition and are dealing with it, there are many stories at every stage throughout the book to give you comfort, hope and inspiration. All the women who are quoted have PCOS. They have shared their stories with us through support group meetings we have attended, conversations over dinner with friends, via email groups and chatrooms, and through direct emails in response to calls we have made at the end of features or flyers in PCOS support group newsletters and meetings. Just so you know where we're coming from too, here are our own PCOS fertility stories to kick things off.

COLETTE'S STORY

'Don't worry, there's a lot they can do nowadays for women who can't have children,' said the ultrasound technician who was scanning me at the appointment I'd fought for months to get.

'What do you mean?' I asked.

'You've got polycystic ovary syndrome,' he said.

'What do you mean?' I repeated blankly.

'I think you'd better ask your doctor about that,' was the reply.

It was December 1996. I was 23 years old, and after months of failing health after coming off the pill — from hair loss to acne, loss of my periods to gaining two stone, fatigue so overwhelming the thought of climbing a flight of stairs made me cry, and mood swings like Jekyll and Hyde — I finally had a diagnosis. I was infertile, and suddenly, for the first time in my life I began to think I wanted children, even though deep down I knew it wasn't the right time.

I had spent months trying to convince my doctors that there was something wrong with me beyond their sense of 'Who doesn't feel tired nowadays?' And here I was, after my doctor sent me for blood tests and a scan but refused to tell me why, being told I couldn't have children and I had polycystic ovary syndrome.

I went back to the doctor clutching my ultrasound scan.

'Congratulations,' he said. I looked at him in confusion.

'Well, you're pregnant I take it?' he said, nodding at the print of the scan in my hand.

'Well, actually I've just found out I can't have children,' I said. And to give him credit he was mightily embarrassed.

Although we hadn't got off to the best of starts, at least he admitted he didn't know anything about PCOS and was happy to refer me to a gynaecologist who he thought might help (the earliest appointment was five months later), but he did reassure me that if I went on the pill to get rid of the symptoms, I could come back when I wanted kids and they'd do their best to sort me out with the miracles of modern medicine. 'There's no reason why you shouldn't be able to have children if you want them,' he said.

Although I was confused, being told one minute I was infertile, and the next that I probably wasn't, my anxiety about whether I wanted to become a mum had been put on hold by his reassurance that there would be options for me if I chose to go down that route. Not only had I never envisaged myself as a mother, having very equivocal feelings about even wanting to have kids at all, I was also in a great but then young relationship (which I'm happily still in now) that was already reeling under the stresses and strains of my hideous PCOS symptoms, on a physical and an emotional level. Why on earth would I want to bring the 'baby or not' question into that mix, either for myself or my partner? It was enough coming to terms with getting a moustache, with bursting into tears at the slightest soppy moment on television or with having breasts so tender and swollen I had to sleep on my back.

Dealing with those symptoms was uppermost in my mind when I decided not just to wait for another five months in misery while I inched up the gynaecologist's waiting list. Instead, I'd turn PCOS detective and see what steps I could be taking myself to deal with the condition. I read everything I could find (not much in 1997 – the internet sites now available, thank goodness, just weren't around then), and talked to doctors, medical herbalists, nutritionists, pharmacists, and other women with PCOS, who I'd been lucky enough to meet through the fledgling UK charity for women with PCOS, Verity. And I began to realize that what I ate, how stressed I was, how much exercise I did, and how much toxic input went into my mind and body could all be having a massive effect on my hormonal balance and insulin resistance.

I made myself a test case and tried a natural healthy eating plan, acupuncture, medical herbalism and nutritional supplements and was astounded with the results – my periods came back within six weeks, the weight started coming off, my painful lumpy spots were reduced massively, my hair loss stopped and my moods evened out. The gynaecologist said I seemed to know more about the condition than she did: 'Whatever you're doing is working really well,' she said, 'I'd suggest you carry on.'

So I did. And I have been doing all this time.

Before I started researching this book, I knew that any woman's fertility starts to decline after 35 and that's there's a lot medical science can offer women with PCOS if they have problems getting pregnant. But now I also know that 70 percent of women with PCOS actually end up getting pregnant naturally, that fertility treatment is thought to be around 90 percent successful for women with PCOS, and that there's a massive amount you can do with your own diet and lifestyle to boost your fertility and the success of any fertility treatment you have. So although I haven't made my choices about motherhood yet, I'm delighted to feel I have choices open to me, and that I can take an active role in managing my own fertility.

Writing this book has been a fascinating journey. I've felt reassured that I'm a woman who just happens to have PCOS, not just a PCOS patient. I'm a woman who has to decide, like any woman, whether motherhood is something I want, and I'm determined not to let my PCOS panic me into making a hasty decision. There's no doubt that having PCOS brings your fertility into sharp focus. But writing this book has helped me see it more clearly than ever – having PCOS doesn't mean you can't have motherhood. In fact, your chances of success are higher than ever now, with more and more research being done (lots of which you'll find in this book), and as it becomes ever more obvious that your diet, stress levels and lifestyle can all have a hugely positive impact. I wish I could find that ultrasound technician and tell him to pass on the good news to anyone else he scans for PCOS!

I sincerely hope this book brings you some information, comfort, inspiration and practical ideas that will help you on your own fertility journey.

THERESA'S STORY

I used to be an energetic person, but everything changed a few months after I stopped taking the pill. I felt as if I was falling apart. I became anxious and moody; it was difficult to concentrate. I was depressed one moment, agitated the next, perpetually tired. Some days even walking up the stairs was exhausting.

After several months of feeling terrible I went to see my doctor. He examined me and assured me I wasn't dying. He asked me when I had had my last period. I told him I hadn't had one since I stopped taking the pill about eight months ago. He told me that I had amenorrhoea. I'd never heard of the word and discovered that it is the medical term used to describe lack of menstruation in women before menopause. I didn't know what to think. Was I going into menopause early?

The doctor explained that many women experience amenorrhea at some point in their lives, especially when they are under stress or after they come off the pill. He asked me if I had been working too hard. He told me to relax and it would sort itself out. He told me to come back in six months. He even joked, saying I should enjoy the freedom of not having a monthly bleed. He suggested going back on the pill, but I told him I didn't want to. I'd only had a few irregular periods before going on the pill in my late teens and I wanted to see if I could menstruate naturally.

My husband assured me that everything would be all right. I appreciated his support, but how could he understand what it felt like to be a woman without her natural rhythms? Having just got married I never knew what to say when friends kept asking when, or if, we were going to start a family. I didn't even have the choice.

I returned in six months to see my doctor. My periods were still absent and my skin was breaking out in spots and blemishes. My hair lacked shine. I looked and felt much older than twenty-eight. I exercised and watched my diet but it was getting harder and harder to keep motivated. My husband was worried. He had never seen me so depressed. The weight was piling on.

This time I was referred for an ultrasound. I was told that there was a slight problem with my ovaries but my doctor said that it was just one of those things and, if I didn't want to start a family right now, there was little point in offering me treatment. Once again he suggested the pill. Once again I refused.

I never had time to think things through as we were due to leave for the United States for a three-year assignment. It was a very exciting time and my health took a backseat while I adjusted to a new way of life. I kept hoping that my periods would return but they never did.

A year or so after we had settled I finally visited a gynaecologist. When I explained that I didn't have periods, I was given progesterone to induce a bleed and told to wait and see if my body could regulate itself and my periods start again. They didn't. By now I was 32 and really starting to think about babies. Even though I had planned on having babies in my mid to late thirties, I could see that time wasn't on my side. Obviously something was wrong.

I was referred to a specialist for a series of tests. The specialist said that I had an excess amount of male hormone circulating in my body, which was interfering with my reproductive cycle, and it was likely I had cysts on my ovaries. An examination confirmed this. I was told that I had polycystic ovaries and as long as I had this condition it could be hard for me to get pregnant. I was told that the condition was very common. I suppose this was meant to make me feel better, but it did not really. I heard the word 'cyst' and imagined the worst. All I thought was 'If the condition is so common why haven't I heard of it? Does this mean I can't have babies?'

Despite feeling anxious I was relieved to finally find out what was wrong and to be taken seriously. Without really knowing what was going on, I agreed to have hormonal treatment: progesterone to encourage a bleed, the fertility drug Clomid to induce ovulation, and hormone injections to release the egg if it was ready. It was an emotional roller coaster of a month when each day seemed the longest ever. The treatment was all I could think about. It was painful and difficult. I had never wanted to have kids so much as I did now. It wasn't easy for my husband either; I shall never forget the look on his face when I'd had my injection and it was suggested that we have intercourse that evening, the following morning, afternoon and evening, and then again the day after. No pressure on the poor guy then!

I jumped for joy when the pregnancy test turned positive after my first attempt. Nine months later I gave birth to a beautiful baby boy. But within a year I was panicking again. I had always planned on two children and my periods hadn't returned. We had now returned to the UK so I visited my doctor again. I was more hopeful this time, as I knew what was wrong with me. I told him I had PCOS and gave him my medical reports from the US. I couldn't believe it when he refused to even look at them and wanted us to go in for basic fertility testing. I didn't want to put either of us through all that again. I decided to change doctor, and thankfully found one who knew about PCOS and was willing to listen. I had the same treatment as before and this time got pregnant after the third attempt. Nine months later I had a beautiful baby girl.

Now that my family was complete, I really turned my attention to my PCOS. A year after my baby girl was born I still wasn't menstruating. I visited three more doctors and all of them suggested the pill, but this wasn't what I wanted. I wanted a natural approach. I did lots of my own research and talked to experts and even wrote a series of articles and a book about hormonal imbalance in women. Then I had a stroke of luck. My editor suggested that I get together with fellow PCOS sufferer, Colette Harris, who had already written a groundbreaking and bestselling book on the subject of PCOS in women. Colette needed a co-author to work with her on *The PCOS Diet Book* – a book designed to encourage women with PCOS to treat their condition through diet, supplements, and exercise and stress relief. This was almost too good to be true. I could write, learn about and treat my condition at the same time.

Over an 18 month period the natural approach has worked brilliantly. My periods have returned naturally and have been as regular as clockwork ever since. I've also got my weight under control and my skin and hair look healthy again. Unless we decide to try for another baby I have no way of knowing if my DIY techniques would have resulted in pregnancy, but I do know that I have never felt healthier and happier. The regularity of my periods indicates a healthy and fertile reproductive cycle. I also think how far I have come from five years ago when I had no idea what was wrong with me and was convinced I'd never have a family of my own. I hope that my experience will give hope and inspiration to every woman diagnosed with PCOS who is concerned about her fertility.

Chapter One
. . . .
What Exactly is PCOS – And How Will it Affect My Fertility?

The key to understanding how and why polycystic ovary syndrome (PCOS) can affect your fertility is to get to grips with what PCOS is. Unfortunately, it's quite a complicated answer, but the basics are that PCOS is a metabolic disorder that can cause hormonal imbalance and a whole menu of symptoms including irregular or absent periods, problems with your fertility, acne, hair loss, weight gain, excess facial hair, diabetes, high blood pressure, fatigue and mood swings. Symptoms can be mild or severe, and your symptoms may not be the same as another women with PCOS – as there are so many symptoms you can end up with a combination that's very particular to you, even if the underlying cause in PCOS cases is the same.

If you've got PCOS you're certainly not alone. Around 10 percent of women have polycystic ovaries, even though many of them may not know it – their symptoms may have been misdiagnosed as PMS or stress, for instance, or they may have PCO which means they have polycystic ovaries on an ultrasound scan but not the symptoms.[4] (When a woman is symptom free, the polycystic ovaries show that she has a built-in predisposition to developing PCOS. If she puts on weight or comes under a great deal of stress she may develop the symptoms.)

THE ROLE OF SEX HORMONES

Often, the imbalance in the sex hormones that are responsible for symptoms like excess hair or acne is also interfering with your ability to ovulate. You can usually tell if you are not ovulating properly by whether or not you're having regular periods, as a 'normal' menstrual cycle involves ovulation followed by a period.

The Normal Menstrual Cycle

In a normal menstrual cycle, the first half, called the follicular phase, starts on the first day of your period and lasts for about 14 days. In this phase the pituitary gland releases low levels of FSH (the follicle-stimulating hormone) to stimulate the follicles in the ovary to ripen their eggs and produce the hormone oestrogen, which causes the lining of the womb to start to thicken in preparation for pregnancy. When levels of oestrogen are high enough the pituitary gland produces a large amount of LH (luteinizing hormone) and the dominant matured follicle in the ovary releases its egg into the fallopian tubes towards the womb in a process called ovulation.

After ovulation comes the second stage of the menstrual cycle, called the luteal phase. Here the cells from the burst follicle collapse to form a cyst called the corpeus luteum. The corpus luteum now produces progesterone as the main hormone of the second half of the cycle. Progesterone causes the thickened lining of the womb to secrete nutrients ready to receive the fertilized egg. If the egg is fertilized it will implant itself in the womb and the corpus luteum will continue to produce progesterone to protect the pregnancy. If it isn't fertilized 14 days after ovulation, the corpus luteum stops producing progesterone and estrogen. The thickened womb lining

starts to break down and is shed as a period, ready for the whole cycle to start again.

If you've got PCOS there is often a problem with the hormones that trigger ovulation every month, which means that not only are irregular or absent periods highly likely but getting pregnant can be harder. On top of that, when ovulation isn't successful you don't get the surge of progesterone to balance the hormone oestrogen in the second half of your cycle which is the normal scheme of things – instead, your oestrogen levels stay the same and can cause symptoms such as bloating, fatigue, absent or irregular periods, hot flushes and dizziness, as well as mood swings and depression.

THE ROLE OF INSULIN

If you have PCOS it's not only your sex hormones that are out of balance and causing ovulation disturbance. Your body's hormonal system, known as the endocrine system, is a web of interconnections, so an imbalance in one hormone can affect the balance of others, too. And in PCOS, insulin is a key hormone that can add to the problem. This is because many women with PCOS are insulin resistant, a condition which makes weight gain easy and weight loss hard – and being overweight can also interfere with your body's ability to ovulate.

Insulin is the hormone that helps cells absorb sugar from the bloodstream. So after a meal, when the blood sugar levels are high and the body wants to store some for energy to use later, the pancreas has to make extra insulin to get the body to store that sugar away. The high surge in insulin means the body goes into sugar storage overdrive and practically clears the bloodstream of any sugar, leading to low blood sugar levels and cravings for more sugary food. This becomes a vicious cycle that can lead to putting on even more weight. If this goes on for years, it can wear out the pancreas's ability to make any more insulin and increase the risk of diabetes.

WHAT ARE THE 'CYSTS'?

High insulin levels also somehow increase the body's output of the sex hormone testosterone, which can cause excess body hair and acne and affect the ovary's ability to mature and release an egg every month. Even though there's usually enough follicle-stimulating hormone (FSH) to encourage your egg follicles to develop, there isn't the right balance of other hormones, such as progesterone or luteinizing hormone (LH) to encourage the egg inside it to mature. And those empty follicles that don't release an egg are the 'cysts' you may have seen on your ultrasound when you were diagnosed.[5] (These cysts are thought to be follicles that have failed to develop completely to release an egg. They are not the same as ovarian cysts, which are normally bigger and found within the ovary.)

These 'cysts', then, are just another symptom of the hormonal imbalances you get when you have PCOS. They are not the cause – and it's interesting to note that in many women who get their diet and lifestyle back on track, or use medication to help deal with their PCOS, the 'cysts' often reduce in size and number in the same way as any other symptom, such as acne, might.

So, PCOS is a metabolic disorder that triggers a series of hormonal imbalances, including raised testosterone, lack of LH and potential insulin resistance, all of which can have an effect on your body's ability to ovulate regularly. And this is how PCOS, and not the 'cysts' on your ovaries, can affect fertility.

What's the difference between PCOS, Syndrome X and Syndrome O?

You may also have heard this group of symptoms described as Syndrome X and Syndrome O.

Syndrome X is a term coined by a group of researchers at Stanford University, to describe a cluster of symptoms, that, when occurring together, increase a person's risk of diabetes, hypertension and heart disease. These symptoms are high blood pressure, insulin resistance, low levels of good cholesterol (HDL) and obesity.

Syndrome O is a term used by reproductive endocrinologist Dr Ronald Feinberg to describe a condition of insulin overproduction and ovarian disruption, which can lead to abnormal bleeding, missed periods, and fertility problems. Feinberg suggests that Syndrome O should replace the term PCOS, as many women with PCOS don't have any significant cysts when checked by ultrasound, although there is still evidence that they may be at risk of developing insulin resistance. He also believes that Syndrome O is easier to teach; most women with PCOS who were polled by the PCOSA desired a name change for the syndrome, recognizing that it is a whole body female problem, not just an ovarian disorder.

Feinberg has a point but on the face of it there really isn't much to distinguish his definition of Syndrome O and the standard definition of PCO and PCOS. It's really just a new name for the cluster of symptoms we recognize as PCOS.

HOW WILL IT AFFECT MY FERTILITY?

However, these symptoms do not mean you're infertile. Infertility means being unable to have a baby when you want one, and as we have seen, 70 percent of women with PCOS conceive naturally. If you've got PCOS and have absent, or irregular periods, or problems with ovulation, you're not infertile – you have a condition known as subfertility. This means that getting pregnant may not be as simple for you as it is for some women but that it's by no means an impossible feat. And it's amazing how much you can do yourself to boost your chances of success.

This is where self-help comes in. A sperm can be a champion swimmer but if ovulation doesn't happen and there is no egg to fertilize, there will be no pregnancy. But in PCOS there are often lots of potential eggs there, just waiting to mature. As the hormonal imbalance of PCOS is the cause of problems with fertility, if you can bring your hormones back into a more regular pattern, you can increase your chances of triggering ovulation. And that's what the information in the fertility-boosting plan in this book is designed to help you do.

HOW WILL IT AFFECT PREGNANCY?

The right hormonal conditions are also essential for a healthy full-term pregnancy. Many of the factors that can upset hormonal balance and hinder fertility or potentially contribute towards miscarriage are within your power to control or change. Simple changes in your diet, lifestyle and attitude can make all the difference. For instance, research suggests that what you eat is very significant for your fertility.[6] Understanding nutrition and correctly supplementing your diet is the first essential step to balancing hormones naturally. Countless studies also show that stress can affect fertility and upset hormonal balance, so managing your stress levels will also help.[7] Weight management problems can also hinder pregnancy and potentially increase the risk of pre-term birth. 'What I try to show my patients with PCOS,' says Dr Robert Franklin, Clinical Professor of Obstetrics and Gynecology at Baylor College of Medicine in Houston, Texas, 'is how her excess or under weight affects her hormones and her ability to get pregnant.' So tackling any weight issues will also boost your chances.

That isn't to say you'll necessarily get pregnant overnight if you eat well, de-stress and deal with weight problems. After all, even 'normal' couples are expected to try for a year before undergoing any medical investigation, and there are other factors you need to bear in mind that may be causing problems with fertility. For example, researchers believe that sperm counts have been reduced by over 40 percent in the last 50 years, with environmental pollutants from plastics and toxins, such as pesticides, thought to inhibit fertility due to their ability to act like oestrogen and disturb hormonal balance.[8] Factors like these show that, far from being something you have little control over, there is a lot you can do to boost your fertility.

WHY DOES IT HAPPEN?

No one is really sure why women with PCOS can't produce the correct balance of hormones so that an ovary can develop and release an egg. There are several theories, including those that suggest that inappropriate levels of the hormones testosterone, insulin, cortisol and LH are the culprits, but the general consensus is that PCOS is most likely a disorder that runs in the family.[9] So if your mum has PCOS and irregular periods, the chances are you will too. Factors such as diet, lifestyle, weight and pollution also contribute to the development of and severity of your symptoms, and although you can't change your genetic heritage, you can change your diet and your lifestyle. You can start to be the driver of your hormonal life to maximize your chances of health and fertility.

Use this book as a practical tool to help boost your fertility levels so your body and mind are in as good a shape as possible for when you do decide to try for a baby, or to help you if you're already trying for one now. And if you're having further problems, the self-help steps throughout the book will also help you get the most from any fertility treatments you may decide to have too.

Chapter Two

. . . .

Your Seven-Step
Fertility-Boosting Action Plan

Getting pregnant isn't just about having sex! Research shows that everything you do in the three or four months before trying to conceive can be as important as the sex itself.[a] What you drink, eat, breathe, do as a job, how stressed you are, how you feel about yourself – everything matters. Any one of them can mean the difference between conceiving and having a healthy baby and not conceiving, especially if you are taking longer to get pregnant than you thought you would.

There is a lot you can do to prepare your body for a healthy pregnancy, and this is what this section of the book is all about. It's an action plan specifically designed for women with PCOS to boost their fertility. The good news is that the great majority of these things are under your control. The even better news is that the self-help approach has helped countless women with PCOS get pregnant and have healthy babies.

HOW TO USE THE PLAN

This PCOS fertility-boosting plan is designed to get you into the best possible shape, both mentally and physically, in order to maximize your chances of conceiving and having a healthy baby. This plan is your basic foundation. You may need nothing more than these seven steps to bring about pregnancy. However, if you're having problems, the seven steps will help your body and mind cope better with overcoming them. If you're having fertility treatment of any kind, the seven steps will enhance the effectiveness of that treatment, as well as your ability to cope with the treatment both physically and emotionally.

In an ideal world we'd recommend that you follow this plan for three to four months before you try to conceive or turn to assisted conception. This is because the healthier you are before you get pregnant or start fertility treatment, the better your chances of conceiving and of the pregnancy resulting in a healthy baby.

World renowned fertility expert, Dr Niels Lauersen, believes: 'While it was once believed that obstetrical treatment should begin only after a conception is confirmed, today most forward thinking physicians recognize that many problems can be prevented when the same care begins before you get pregnant.' This concept is known as preconceptual care, a programme of healthy living for you and your partner that will boost your chances of fertility.

THE IMPORTANCE OF PRECONCEPTUAL CARE

Many fertility specialists now recommend preconception care whenever a couple decides that they want to start a family, and this has particular benefits for women with PCOS. Research on women with PCOS has shown how effective diet and lifestyle change can be for the condition, and how it can not only improve symptoms such as irregular periods, weight gain, acne and facial hair, but also dramatically increase your chances of both conception and a healthy full-term pregnancy.[10-13]

Whether you are about to try for a baby the first time, or are at the stage where you're considering fertility drugs, the action plan is a good idea. Not only might you get a surprise natural pregnancy (the National Institute of Environmental Health Sciences in North Carolina showed that couples who failed to conceive naturally within the first year did conceive naturally in the second year[b]), you will also enhance the power of the fertility treatment itself. 'After alteration in lifestyle,' says PCOS expert Dr Samuel Thatcher, 'some women with PCOS can avoid ever being seen in a fertility clinic.'

YOUR FOUR-MONTH PRECONCEPTION PLAN

Even when your future baby is still a longing or a twinkle in your eye, you and your partner can both be taking steps towards a healthy conception. The healthier you both are, the better your chances of conceiving sooner rather than later, and of the pregnancy producing a healthy baby at the end.

Why Four Months?

Three to four months is the recommended period of time for preconceptual care because it takes about three months for a new batch of sperm to be made and three months for a woman's egg to develop from its follicle and be released. It also takes between six weeks and three months to eliminate certain toxins from your system properly, and to raise the level of crucial fertility-boosting nutrients in your blood serum. Research spearheaded by Foresight and backed up by UK doctors suggests that a good three- to four-month programme of healthy living will maximize your chances of conception, whether you want to try now, or in the future.[14]

Taking care of yourself before you get pregnant is not only important for your fertility – it's crucial for your baby-to-be too. The egg that is released at conception is the product of your diet and lifestyle, and experts now believe that what a woman eats prior to conception is just as significant to the health of the baby as what she eats during pregnancy.[15]

According to Irwin Emanuel MD, Professor of Epidemiology and Pediatrics at the University of Washington in Seattle, 'If you are undernourished your baby could well become "programmed" at conception to develop high blood pressure, clotting disorders, abnormal glucose, insulin and cholesterol problems and even hormonal problems like PCOS.'

The first weeks of pregnancy are increasingly understood to be the most important in terms of fetal development as all the major organs – heart, lungs, liver, kidneys, nervous system – are all formed then. Remember, women are already two weeks pregnant before they miss a period, so eating well in the run up to a pregnancy is really important.

YOUR SEVEN STEPS TO FERTILITY

Every woman with PCOS is unique and there is no one magic formula that will work for all, but making healthy diet and lifestyle choices before you get pregnant can yield dramatic results. For at least three months before trying to conceive you (and your partner) should:

1. Manage your weight.

2. Get as fit and as well as you can.

3. Reduce the level of stress in your life.

4. Eat fresh, healthy food and make sure you get your pro-fertility nutrients.

5. Detox your diet and your lifestyle to get rid of anti-fertility chemicals.

6. Ask yourself if you are ready

7. Enjoy your sex life

WHY YOUR PARTNER NEEDS TO FOLLOW THE SEVEN STEPS

A good preconceptual care programme involves getting both partners into the best possible physical and mental shape before trying for a baby. In couples with fertility problems, it is thought that approximately one-third can be attributed to the male partner, one-third to the female partner and one-third to a combination of both partners. For couples who are having difficulty getting pregnant, doing all the seven steps to fertility together is important because, although your baby will be nourished inside you, it takes both your egg and your partner's sperm to make a baby.

If both partners are physically and emotionally fit, the healthier your eggs or sperm are and the better your chances of getting and staying pregnant. Never lose sight of the fact that getting pregnant takes two and there may be other problems aside from PCOS. If you are not as fertile as you could be owing to irregular ovulation, and your partner has lower than normal sperm count, this can reduce your chances even further.

For men the most common problem is not just how many sperm there are but sperm quality. In other words, are they strong and fit enough to reach and penetrate a ripe egg? Both sperm quality and quantity can be affected by lifestyle factors, such as poor diet, stress, too little exercise, smoking and alcohol. In addition, your partner should avoid hot baths, tight underpants, exposure to heat, traffic fumes, mobile phones, and long hours sitting and driving. Why? Because studies have shown that all these factors can have a negative effect on sperm quality and quantity.[16] This gives a man a great deal of control over his own fertility, and numerous studies have shown that simple diet and lifestyle changes can improve sperm in as little as three months.[17]

STEP ONE: MANAGE YOUR WEIGHT

'About a year ago I was diagnosed with PCOS and told that if I wanted to start a family it might be harder than I thought. I was told that I'd improve my chances if I lost some weight. It was a shock and at first I felt completely overwhelmed. Steve and I had been trying for a baby for a while now and this wasn't good news. As for losing weight, I'd been trying for years and had tried every diet in the book so how was I going to manage it now? My doctor referred me to a dietician who had treated women with PCOS before. I was given advice about healthy food choices and encouraged to take up some gentle exercise – so I started walking to work instead of taking the bus. Within four months I had gone down two dress sizes, my periods got regular and my acne improved. I felt wonderful for the first time in years. Then about a year after being diagnosed, when I was just about to go back to my doctor for fertility treatment something amazing happened – I fell pregnant.'

CHARLOTTE, 33

Your Ideal Body Weight

Carrying too much body fat can make symptoms of PCOS – including irregular periods – worse, and stop you getting pregnant. Losing weight, if you have weight to lose, can improve symptoms and boost your fertility. So if you have PCOS and are concerned about fertility, being around the right weight for your height could prove crucial. Your ideal weight for health and fertility is determined by your body mass index, or BMI. A BMI between 21 and 25 is perfect and between 23 and 24 ideal for conception. The average woman has 27 percent of her weight as body fat.

Body Mass Index Table

BMI	Normal						Overweight					Obese										Extreme Obesity														
	19	20	21	22	23	24	25	26	27	28	29	30	31	32	33	34	35	36	37	38	39	40	41	42	43	44	45	46	47	48	49	50	51	52	53	54
Height (inches)	Body Weight (pounds)																																			
58	91	96	100	105	110	115	119	124	129	134	138	143	148	153	158	162	167	172	177	181	186	191	196	201	205	210	215	220	224	229	234	239	244	248	253	258
59	94	99	104	109	114	119	124	128	133	138	143	148	153	158	163	168	173	178	183	188	193	198	203	208	212	217	222	227	232	237	242	247	252	257	262	267
60	97	102	107	112	118	123	128	133	138	143	148	153	158	163	168	174	179	184	189	194	199	204	209	215	220	225	230	235	240	245	250	255	261	266	271	276
61	100	106	111	116	122	127	132	137	143	148	153	158	164	169	174	180	185	190	195	201	206	211	217	222	227	232	238	243	248	254	259	264	269	275	280	285
62	104	109	115	120	126	131	136	142	147	153	158	164	169	175	180	186	191	196	202	207	213	218	224	229	235	240	246	251	256	262	267	273	278	284	289	295
63	107	113	118	124	130	135	141	146	152	158	163	169	175	180	186	191	197	203	208	214	220	225	231	237	242	248	254	259	265	270	278	282	287	293	299	304
64	110	116	122	128	134	140	145	151	157	163	169	174	180	186	192	197	204	209	215	221	227	232	238	244	250	256	262	267	273	279	285	291	296	302	308	314
65	114	120	126	132	138	144	150	156	162	168	174	180	186	192	198	204	210	216	222	228	234	240	246	252	258	264	270	276	282	288	294	300	306	312	318	324
66	118	124	130	136	142	148	155	161	167	173	179	186	192	198	204	210	216	223	229	235	241	247	253	260	266	272	278	284	291	297	303	309	315	322	328	334
67	121	127	134	140	146	153	159	166	172	178	185	191	198	204	211	217	223	230	236	242	249	255	261	268	274	280	287	293	299	306	312	319	325	331	338	344
68	125	131	138	144	151	158	164	171	177	184	190	197	203	210	216	223	230	236	243	249	256	262	269	276	282	289	295	302	308	315	322	328	335	341	348	354
69	128	135	142	149	155	162	169	176	182	189	196	203	209	216	223	230	236	243	250	257	263	270	277	284	291	297	304	311	318	324	331	338	345	351	358	365
70	132	139	146	153	160	167	174	181	188	195	202	209	216	222	229	236	243	250	257	264	271	278	285	292	299	306	313	320	327	334	341	348	355	362	369	376
71	136	143	150	157	165	172	179	186	193	200	208	215	222	229	236	243	250	257	265	272	279	286	293	301	308	315	322	329	338	343	351	358	365	372	379	386
72	140	147	154	162	169	177	184	191	199	206	213	221	228	235	242	250	258	265	272	279	287	294	302	309	316	324	331	338	346	353	361	368	375	383	390	397
73	144	151	159	166	174	182	189	197	204	212	219	227	235	242	250	257	265	272	280	288	295	302	310	318	325	333	340	348	355	363	371	378	386	393	401	408
74	148	155	163	171	179	186	194	202	210	218	225	233	241	249	256	264	272	280	287	295	303	311	319	326	334	342	350	358	365	373	381	389	396	404	412	420
75	152	160	168	176	184	192	200	208	216	224	232	240	248	256	264	272	279	287	295	303	311	319	327	335	343	351	359	367	375	383	391	399	407	415	423	431
76	156	164	172	180	189	197	205	213	221	230	238	246	254	263	271	279	287	295	304	312	320	328	336	344	353	361	369	377	385	394	402	410	418	426	435	443

Source: Adapted from *Clinical Guidelines on the Identification, Evaluation, and Treatment of Overweight and Obesity in Adults: The Evidence Report.*

Source: the National Heart, Lung and Blood Institute.

Why Weight Is Important for Fertility

A certain amount of body fat is vital to maintain your menstrual cycle. Fat is essential to fertility as women need body fat in order to ovulate. Young girls do not begin their periods until they are at least 17 percent body fat. Studies have shown that 50 percent of women who have a BMI (Body Mass Index) below 20.7 are infertile.[18]

If your BMI is lower than 20 you may want to delay trying for a baby until you adjust your diet to give your body the resources it needs. Low body weight and sudden weight loss due to a poor diet can disrupt hormonal balance and stop you ovulating – think of it as nature's way of preventing conception when mom isn't properly nourished. Having said that, women who are underweight or eating poorly do conceive, but these women face a higher risk of miscarriage or giving birth to a baby who is underweight or premature. Infants with low birth weight are vulnerable to infection and prone to feeding problems in the early weeks of life.

However, you can have too much of a good thing. Statistics for 2002 from the UK's Office for National Statistics show that over half of all British women are either overweight or clinically obese, having a BMI over 30. Being overweight can interfere with ovulation because the extra fat produces extra oestrogen in your system, causing an imbalance in the ratio of the reproductive hormones needed for egg development and release.

If your BMI is outside the fertile range we recommend that you delay trying to get pregnant until you find ways to manage the situation (see our PCOS weight loss and gain tips, below). We don't recommend dieting. Dieting for weight loss or eating the wrong kinds of food for weight gain can mean that you aren't giving your body the nutrients it needs to ovulate regularly and stay healthy.

We know that both PCOS and obesity increase the risk of infertility but thankfully the effect is quickly reversed.[19–21] Even losing a small amount of weight can be enough to stimulate ovulation again and make periods regular.[22] A study by the University of Adelaide in 1995 involved 12 overweight women who were not ovulating.[23,24] After following a six-month programme of diet and exercise, 11 of them conceived naturally. Another study by the University of Milan in 2003 involved 33 overweight women with PCOS who lost 5 percent of their body weight.[25] Ten pregnancies occurred, 15 experienced spontaneous ovulation and 18 had a resumption of regular cycles.

If you've got PCOS and think you're overweight, don't panic! Your ideal weight for fertility is probably a good deal heavier than you think.

The ideal body weight for a woman's fertility covers a wide range but, if you are at the low or high end of the range, this can increase the chances of irregular periods without ovulation. This is a known as anovulation – and when no egg is released you can't get pregnant.

How Weight Affects PCOS Symptoms

Research shows that not only are women with PCOS more likely to be overweight but that being overweight makes symptoms of PCOS worse, especially fertility problems.[23,26,27] If you have PCOS, in addition to your body's typical reaction to restricted food intake (that is, your body goes into starvation mode and your metabolism, the rate at which your body uses the calories or energy from food, slows so that you reach a point when even though you are eating less you can't lose weight), you have another hurdle to face. It has been shown that women with PCOS actually store fat more efficiently and burn calories more slowly than women who don't have PCOS.[28] You're in a catch-22 situation. Your inability to lose weight can lead to comfort eating, so you end up feeling trapped in a vicious cycle with the pounds piling on.

But don't lose heart – even with PCOS, you can regain control of the situation. For women with PCOS the best way to lose weight isn't to diet, but simply to eat healthily and increase your amount of exercise. This helps you control your blood sugar levels to reduce cravings for sugary foods, as well as helping you burn off more calories. 'Of utmost importance to a patient with PCOS who has weight to lose' says Dr Robert Franklin, Professor of Obstetrics and Gynecology at Baylor College of Medicine in Houston, Texas 'is her realization that fast or fad diets will not help – she must follow a diet and exercise program that she can live with for the rest of her life.' If you feel as if you just don't know where to start, visit your doctor. Simple weight-loss advice from a physician and regular follow-up helped obese women with polycystic ovary syndrome lose a substantial amount of weight, revealed a recent study presented to The Endocrine Society by Lysanne Pelletier, MD, a trainee at the University of Sherbrooke.[30]

Your PCOS Weight Loss Guidelines

- The basic rule is to burn off more calories than you take in, so you need to exercise regularly!

- Aim for a slow, gradual weight loss of no more than 2lbs a week. It may not sound much but it soon adds up. Aim to get into your ideal weight range, not at the bottom of it.

- Include more fresh fruits and vegetables in your diet. Remember a glass of diluted fresh pressed juice, or frozen vegetables, count too.

- Eat healthy, fresh, preferably organic food – it only takes 10 minutes to whip up a stir fry, a bowl of crunchy salad or a home-made soup.

- Get into the habit of snacking on healthy foods throughout the day to keep your blood sugar levels on an even keel. Start your day with a good breakfast, have a healthy mid-morning snack – such as an apple and a couple of almonds – followed by lunch, a mid-afternoon snack – such as carrot sticks with a low fat cheese dip – and a light supper.

- Don't eat big meals after 8 p.m.

- Limit your intake of animal and dairy fats. Only eat lean, grilled meats and low-fat dairy foods.

- Try to drink at least six to eight glasses of fresh water a day. And drink a couple before each meal, if you want to enhance your weight loss, says the latest randomized, controlled trial from Virginia Tech in

Blacksburg, Virginia, USA, published by The American Chemical Society, 2010. 'In this recent study, we found that over the course of 12 weeks, dieters who drank water before meals, three times per day, lost about 5 pounds more than dieters who did not increase their water intake,' says Brenda Davy, PhD, lead author. The researchers suggested water may be so effective simply because it fills up the stomach with a substance that has zero calories, reducing appetite. Increased water consumption may also help people lose weight if they drink it in place of sweetened calorie-containing beverages, said Davy.[31]

- Limit your intake of sugar, sweets, cakes, biscuits, salt, alcohol and caffeine, and foods high in chemicals, additives and preservatives, such as many ready-made meals or tinned produce.

- Increase your intake of fibre by eating more fruit and veg, with cereals such as muesli, and by choosing brown rice, bread and pasta.

- Eat good quality protein (lean meats, skimmed dairy products, nuts and seeds) with every meal.

- Aim to eat fish at least twice a week and nuts and seeds (flax, sunflower, hemp, walnuts, cashews) daily.

- Watch your portion size – if you have PCOS your body stores more calories from the food you do eat, and it's amazing how much less your body needs than your appetite wants.

- Chew thoroughly and put your knife and fork down between each mouthful – taking time means that you'll feel fuller more quickly.

- Remember the 80/20 rule. You can't eat healthily all the time and the occasional treat – a bar of chocolate or bag of chips – doesn't mean that you have failed. It is the excesses that are dangerous. It is important that you enjoy your food and allow yourself the occasional indulgence. So no food is off limit.

- Do more exercise so you can eat plenty of nutritious food but still lose weight: it can be a brisk 20-minute walk every day to start with, as long as you start doing more than you are doing now. Exercise is really key if you have PCOS, so you need to get motivated and stay motivated to do it. Try finding an exercise buddy to keep you going, consider a personal trainer to kick-start your programme, or get your partner to come with you for regular walks where you can talk about the day as you exercise.

- If your partner has weight to lose, encourage him to lose it too. Being overweight can affect male fertility and reduce the quality and quantity of his sperm count.[32]

- If you find that you need more advanced weight loss help, or feel that emotional eating is your underlying issue, turn to our next chapter on tackling stubborn problems for more ideas (see page 91).

Beat Belly Fat

Research shows that fat around the middle – known as abdominal or visceral fat – puts us at a higher risk of diabetes, high blood pressure and fatty liver disease. Believe it or not, recent research has also linked it to an increased risk of depression and osteoporosis.[33,34] So if you put on weight around your middle (typically an 'apple' shape instead of a 'pear' shape), here are some extra ideas to help you shift it.

- *Eat soluble fibre, and exercise:* For every 10 g increase in soluble fibre eaten per day, visceral fat was reduced by 3.7 percent over five years, in participants, says recent research from Wake Forest Baptist Medical Center. That means eat more soluble fibre from vegetables, fruit and beans – 10 g of soluble fibre can be achieved by eating two small apples, one cup of green peas and one-half cup of pinto beans. In addition, increased moderate activity resulted in a 7.4 percent decrease in the rate of visceral fat accumulation over the same time period – moderate activity means exercising vigorously for 30 minutes, two to four times a week.

- *Enjoy blueberries:* Eating more of these antioxidant-rich berries could help reduce the likelihood of laying down belly fat, says recent research using rats in a laboratory.[35] More research is needed in humans, but if you're eating five-a-day anyway, where's the harm in making blueberries part of the mix?

- *Keep exercising after weight loss:* A study conducted by exercise physiologists in the University of Alabama at Birmingham (UAB) Department of Human Studies found that as little as 80 minutes a week of aerobic or resistance training helps not only to prevent weight gain, but also to inhibit a regain of harmful visceral fat one year after weight loss.[36]

- *Reduce stress, boost nutrition:* Nutritionist Dr Marilyn Glenville PhD, author of *Fat Around the Middle*, recommends shifting this weight by reducing your body's stress response, a process that pushes your body to store fat around your abdomen. Taking a good quality multivitamin and mineral that includes stressbusting vitamin B6, magnesium, zinc and biotin; eating more omega-3 essential fats from oily fish, linseeds, walnuts, soya, pumpkin seeds and green leafy vegetables; reducing sugar and white flour products such as white bread will all help, she says.

PCOS Weight Gain Guidelines

If weight gain, not weight loss, is a factor, don't be tempted to reach for biscuits and unhealthy junk food in order to increase your calorie intake. Try to resist these foods as they fill you up and will prevent you eating the more nutritious fertility-boosting foods that your body and your future baby-to-be needs. Aim to eat little and often and consume plenty of healthy, fresh foods – especially fruits and vegetables and food rich in oils, such as fish, nuts, seeds and olives.

Weight Loss Tips from a PCOS Nutrition Specialist

21st century lifestyles mean it's easier to put on weight than ever before, so here's how to take back control, says NHS senior dietitian Bernice Chiswell, who runs a PCOS weight loss clinic at Bedford Hospital, UK.

If you have PCOS and are finding it hard to lose weight, it's interesting to know we live in what's called an 'obesogenic environment'. Compared to our grandparents' generation we're less active, with more people owning cars, using labour-saving devices, having less physically demanding jobs, and spending more leisure time in front of a screen. On top of this we're eating more fast food, larger portions, and snacking on high fat high, sugar foods and drinks. No wonder we are getting fatter as a nation, with nearly a quarter of the population obese. (Check out the eye opening quizzes at hp2010.nhlbihin.net/portion). This means today's lifestyles tend to lead to weight gain, unless we make conscious decisions to buck the trend.

The Good News

If you are very overweight (Body Mass Index of 30 or more) then the good news is that just a 5-10% weight loss can:

- Reduce the excess insulin
- Regulate periods
- Reduce acne and unwanted hair growth
- Halve your risk of developing diabetes
- Improve blood pressure and cholesterol levels
- Reduce the risk of heart disease, strokes and certain cancers
- Reduce pressure on joints e.g. knees and back
- Increase length and quality of life

So, for example, if you weigh 100 kg or 15 ½ stone, aim to reach 90 kg (14 ¼ stone). With an average loss of 1kg (2lbs) a week, this may only take 10 weeks! Beware of programmes that promote quick weight loss. A lot of people who lose weight very quickly find they put it back on very quickly, too (and even go beyond their original weight), in a phenomenon known as yo-yoing, which can compromise your health.

Prepare for Success

There is no 'one way' which is right for everyone. But to get you inspired, here are some tips from the American National Weight Control Registry, which includes over 5,000 members (80% are women) who have lost at least 30 lbs (over 2 stone) and kept it off for a year or more (check out www.nwcr.ws for some of their inspirational stories).

- 45% lost weight on their own; 55% lost weight with some type of programme.
- 98% modified their food intake.
- 94% increased physical activity, the most frequently reported form of activity being walking.
- 90% exercise about 1 hour daily on average (*tip*: as well as helping lose weight and keep it off, being more active burns up the extra insulin so can reduce PCOS symptoms).
- 78% eat breakfast every day.
- 75% weigh themselves at least once a week (*tip*: don't check your weight too often while trying to lose as it will fluctuate daily, which can be de-motivating).
- Most report keeping weight off by continuing to maintain a low calorie, low fat diet and doing high levels of activity.
- 62% watch less than 10 hours TV weekly.

And an additional insight from Professor Adam Balen which will make you feel better if you're not one for sticking to a specific diet regime: 'Any diet that is sustainable is a good thing. Low GI has some logic but evidence is that there is not a PCOS diet despite all that is written about it.'

If you really hate to exercise and hate gym, sport or classes why not take up walking? Walking is ideal, as it doesn't really seem like exercise, but even 10 or 15 minutes a day can make a real difference. In fact, walking is highly recommended for women with PCOS. Dr Robert Franklin believes that, 'Walking is particularly good for PCOS patients. Not only is it great exercise but it is a great way to

de-stress and give you some time to yourself.'

Note: **For all of the above activities, start slowly and don't push yourself too hard. You should always consult your doctor before starting any new exercise programme.**

STEP TWO: GET AS FIT AND AS WELL AS YOU CAN

Becoming as fit and as well as you possibly can involves both you and your partner exercising regularly, as well as getting the all clear from your GP and getting checked for and treating any infections.

The Benefits of Exercise

For women with PCOS exercise is particularly beneficial. Not only can it kick-start weight loss but it has also been proven to help insulin and glucose control, which in turn means your ovaries are encouraged to produce less testosterone, promote hormonal balance, and so ease symptoms. Also when symptoms of PCOS result in loss of self-esteem, exercise can help you feel good about yourself, and when you feel good, you're less likely to eat unhealthy foods, and more likely to feel positive towards your fertility-boosting plan.

Exercise can also boost fertility. You don't have to be fit to be fertile but it sure can help. If you are reasonably fit, this can improve your chances of conceiving. Regular exercise can regulate your hormones and menstrual cycle in a beneficial way by helping you reach a healthy body weight and keeping stress levels down, therefore encouraging regular ovulation.[37]

Don't overdo it though. Training for more than 15 hours a week will have the opposite effect and inhibit ovulation.[38] Women who exercise to the extreme, such as gymnasts and dancers and athletes, can lose their menstrual cycle because of the reduction in body weight. Exercise has lots of other benefits too for you and your partner. For example:

- it reduces stress

- lowers blood sugar levels

- promotes insulin efficiency

- promotes good sleep patterns

- boosts circulation

- reduces the risk of heart disease and diabetes

- improves blood supply to your reproductive organs

- boosts your feeling of both mental and physical wellbeing.

With all these benefits, small wonder that fitter people tend to feel more confident and sexy.[39, c]

Fitting Exercise into Your Life

A good, balanced exercise programme provides three important benefits: stamina, strength and flexibility. A woman needs all three to lift and carry a baby, run after a small child, and cope with the day-to-day stresses of motherhood. Plus, getting in shape at least three months before you conceive may make it easier to maintain an active lifestyle during pregnancy and actually enjoy those nine months, not to mention helping you to get through labour.

Strengthening your back muscles now, for example, can stave off lower back pain later, and aerobic exercise can improve your mood and energy levels, not to mention help you achieve a healthy pre-pregnancy weight. You'll also be less vulnerable to the hormonal shifts that can make pregnant women irritable and send family and friends running for cover.

Great exercises to help get into shape for pregnancy include running, power walking and jogging, swimming, cycling and aerobics. Some of these are fairly strenuous, however, and should not be taken up for the first time while pregnant, so be sure to begin well before you start trying to conceive. Then you can continue your routine when you're pregnant. For flexibility and stress relief, exercises such as tai chi, yoga and pilates are also good.

How Fit Are You?

TEST YOURSELF:

Can you walk briskly for ten minutes without feeling exhausted?

Can you walk up a flight of stairs without losing your breath?

Sit quietly and check your resting pulse rate. Find your pulse where your wrist joins your hand, just below the thumb and about 1cm from the edge of your wrists. Count the beats for 20 seconds then multiply by three. If the results are under 70 you are pretty fit, 80–100 is okay (ish), over 100 isn't okay, and is a sign that you need to get fit.

Aim for around 30 minutes of continuous exercise that works the large muscles and elevates your breathing and heart rate every day, or every other day. If you're a beginner, start with 10 minutes and gradually build to 30 minutes over a period of three to four months. Fitting exercise into your life is much easier if you find something you enjoy. Check out what your fitness options are. Could you walk to work instead of drive? How about taking up running or joining a fitness class? Do you enjoy swimming or cycling? Or would you enjoy something else. Jive dancing? Yoga? Martial arts? And don't forget the latest trends that make exercise feel like more fun, from boxing classes, to zumba, belly dancing to mall walking (power walking around a shopping mall with an organised group – great for winter!). Ask your friends and work colleagues what they do, and check out the timetables at your local gym or sports centre.

VISIT YOUR DOCTOR FOR A GENERAL CHECKUP

If you do want to try for a baby it is important that you visit your doctor for a general checkup. This needs to include the following:

- Blood pressure test

- Urine check for infection and also for blood sugar levels

- A cervical smear

- A blood group test

- A discussion of any long-term health conditions, such as diabetes, and their implications for pregnancy

- A discussion of any medication you are taking to see if it is safe to take during pregnancy, and that it will not affect your fertility

- An investigation for silent genitourinary (GU) infections that could affect your chances of getting pregnant. You may not even know that you have one, as in some cases there are no noticeable symptoms. Ideally, before you try to get pregnant you and your partner should have a screen test at a GU clinic for infections such as: chlamydia, trichomoniasis, mycoplasma and ureaplasma, HIV, CMV, rubella, Group B haemolytic streptococci, gardnerella and toxoplasmois. Your partner should also be tested for toxoplasmosis and cytomegalovirus, which, although not GU infections, can also play havoc with fertility. If the sperm is infected even mildly, it can make all the difference between being able to help make a baby and not.

YOUR GENERAL HEALTH

The preconception period is the ideal time to really focus on your general health and wellbeing. Do you wake up in the morning feeling energetic or do you crawl out of bed feeling exhausted before the day has begun? Do you rarely get ill or are you always going down with colds and infections? Is it easy for you to get around or do you suffer from fatigue and/or mysterious aches and pains which slow you down? If it's the latter, these could be signs that your health isn't at optimum level. Eating healthily and exercising regularly may be all that you need to get you back on track, but if you don't feel as fit and as well as you possibly can, do discuss this with your doctor.

THE AGE ISSUE

Are you over 35? The medical term for the mature mum (any woman who has a baby over the age of 30) is quite intimidating: elderly primigravida. Although more and more women are having babies later in life, it is important to bear in mind that the 20s are considered to be our reproductive prime, with the least amount of fertility and health complications for mother and child.

Whether you have PCOS or not, at about the age of 35 most

women start to become less fertile and may not ovulate every month, even though they still menstruate regularly. (A slight shortening of the monthly menstrual cycle is also common with age.) If you have PCOS and are having problems ovulating, clearly being over 35 isn't going to boost your chances, but try not to let this panic you. You can still raise your fertility levels with diet, exercise, health checks and, if necessary, fertility treatment.

CONTRACEPTION

You may be wondering why we're discussing contraception in a book about fertility! While you're getting as fit and as well as you can before trying to conceive, you need to use a form of contraception you can trust, but which will also allow your fertility to return quickly when you stop using it. If you have PCOS what are your options?

The Combined Pill

The combined pill is one of the most reliable forms of contraception and the treatment most likely to be offered by your doctor for PCOS symptoms such as irregular periods, acne and hair loss, but what are the pros and cons when it comes to the effect on your fertility?

Studies have shown that it could cause a number of nutrient deficiencies, including vitamin B1, B2, B6 and B12, vitamin C and E, zinc and folic acid.[40] As you'll see in step four, below, all of these are essential fertility-boosting nutrients. Or you could ensure that you make changes in your diet and lifestyle to counteract the problems the pill can cause. Women with PCOS who are on the pill need more than ever to eat healthily and exercise regularly and to take a good multivitamin and mineral to avoid nutritional deficiencies.

According to the British Medical Association Concise Guide to

Medicine and Drugs, the pill can also affect blood sugar balance: 'Estrogens may also trigger the onset of diabetes mellitus in susceptible women, or aggravate blood-sugar control in diabetic women.[41] This isn't good news for women with PCOS since the condition is already associated with insulin resistance (a precursor state to diabetes).[42] High levels of insulin stimulate the ovaries to produce large amounts of male hormones called androgens. Excess androgens are thought to stop the ovaries releasing an egg, causing irregular or absent periods and subfertility.

When the pill first came on the market there was much concern about its long-term threat to fertility but so far that is a concern that remains unproven, and most women ovulate within six to eight weeks when they withdraw from it. Indeed, there are some studies that suggest that the pill can actually boost fertility, with some research suggesting that by preventing ovulation it preserves your better quality eggs for future use later on.[43]

The official advice from the National Health Service in the UK is as follows: it takes a while for your periods to come back after you stop taking the pill. For most women, it's 2 to 4 weeks before you have a period, but this depends on the individual and what your cycle is normally like. Weight, health, stress, exercise and conditions such as polycystic ovary syndrome can all influence the cycle of periods.

Your periods may be irregular when you first come off the pill, and you should allow up to six months for your natural cycle to re-establish itself fully. It's quite common to have a longer delay before normal periods start again after stopping the pill, especially if you have run two or three packets together. This is because the pill contains the hormones that stop ovulation (the release of an egg) each month.

There appears to be no connection between how long the pill has been taken and having fertility problems. Some women conceive immediately after stopping taking the pill. While the pill doesn't cause fertility problems, it does mask problems that were already there, such as irregular periods.

As soon as you come off the pill, you can get pregnant. It's therefore important to use another form of contraception, such as condoms, straightaway.

If you're trying to get pregnant, it's a good idea to wait to have one natural period first. This gives you time to make sure you are in the best of health for pregnancy, for example, by starting to take folic acid supplements and quitting smoking. It also helps your GP or midwife to predict your due date accurately.[44]

Other pill studies, however, give a different picture of the pill's effect on fertility and the significance of this for women with PCOS.[45–47] Some studies suggest that among previously fertile women who stop taking the pill in order to conceive, the majority delivered a child within 30 months. These statistics seem to bode well but it was found in another study of 'older' childless women, aged between 30 and 35, that they experienced a marked delay in conceiving when coming off the pill: 50 percent of these women took a year longer to get pregnant – sometimes taking as long as 72 months – than those of the same age who had not been using the pill. Few women – and much less ones over 35 with PCOS – want to risk waiting six years once they start trying for a baby. More to the point, the study only looked at 30- to 35-year-olds; there have been no similar studies on women older than this and logic would indicate that the figures probably wouldn't get better, but worse. Now add PCOS into the mix – a condition which further reduces your chances of conceiving – and the picture becomes quite a gloomy one.

So should you take the pill? The choice, of course, is yours, but the chance that you could be one of those women who experience a long delay in conceiving once you come off it would seem to suggest that switching to a more natural form of contraception as part of your preconceptual care routine is a good idea. If you are concerned, you might want to discuss with your doctor other contraceptive methods or other treatments for irregular periods, hair loss, facial or body hair, or acne.

The Progesterone-Only Pill

The progesterone-only pill works by thickening the cervical mucous so that sperm can't get to the egg. If you miss a single dose, fertility can return within two days and there isn't any evidence of a delay in fertility once you stop using it. However, some women with PCOS say that the progesterone-only pill makes symptoms worse, and a study at the University of Southern California Medical School found that the progestin-only pill increased the risk of insulin resistance and diabetes.[48]

Contraceptive Injections and Hormone Implants

Contraceptive injections such as Dep-Provera and Noristerat, and implants offer protection for anything between eight and twelve weeks for injections, and up to three years for implants. They work by stopping ovulation and making your womb lining thinner and less likely to accept a fertilized egg. Your fertility and periods may take several months or years to return, even if you only ever had one injection or implant, and for this reason they aren't the most sensible choice for women with PCOS.

The IUD (Intrauterine Device)

The IUD is 98 percent effective, depending on which type is used. It is a small plastic device that works by causing a mild inflammation of the womb so its lining will not allow a fertilized egg to implant. An IUD will also inhibit the sperm's ability to move. Fertility usually returns promptly after an IUD removal, but it is important that you are aware that there is always a risk of it causing pelvic infection while it is in place. If such an infection were to reach your fallopian tube and cause scarring, the blockage could affect your future fertility.

Barrier Methods

Barrier methods of contraception include the diaphragm, cervical cap, condom and female condoms. They work by stopping sperm from reaching the small passageway that runs through the centre of the cervix. If used with spermicides, which work by killing sperm, they are approximately 97 percent effective.

Barrier methods are probably the best choice of contraception for women with a hormonal problem like PCOS, as they don't involve hormonal manipulation. In addition, your fertility will return as soon as you stop using them, which makes them the ideal choice of contraception for a couple following a preconceptual care programme.

NATURAL FAMILY PLANNING

By learning to recognize your fertile time of the month you can work out when to have intercourse to maximize or minimize your chances of pregnancy. This is the theory behind natural family planning (NFP).

With NFP you time intercourse to coincide with ovulation if you want to get pregnant, and avoid it when you are ovulating if you don't. There are only a few days in each cycle when an egg is ripe for fertilization. A cycle is the time between the start of one period and the start of the next. To count the days of a cycle, start with the first day of the menstrual bleeding: this is day one. Continue counting until the first day of the next bleed, when you return to day one. An average cycle lasts around 28 days, although anything between 21 and 35 days is considered normal.

In a regular 28-day cycle ovulation will normally take place around days 12–14 before the next period. There are various schools of thought, but it is generally held that if a couple is trying to get pregnant they should make love at least every other day around ovulation. Sperm are capable of fertilizing an egg up to 48 hours after ejaculation, some even longer, and an egg can be fertilized for up to 24 hours after ovulation. This gives a window of around three to six days in the cycle during which intercourse should take place if you want to get pregnant, or be avoided if you don't.

If you do have regular menstrual cycles, keep a record over a period of months so that you can assess those days when ovulation is most likely to occur, by subtracting 14 from your expected start date. There is some variation, but most doctors suggest that, if you have a 28-day cycle, your fertile week would run from day 10 to 17.

This all sounds so simple but in reality it isn't. It's fine if your periods are regular, but what if you can't really predict your fertile week because your cycles change all the time? Most women don't have completely regular cycles, and the majority of women with PCOS have irregular or absent cycles – even if periods do occur regularly this is not necessarily a definite indication of ovulation. If your periods are absent, NFP obviously isn't for you (see Chapter Three: Tackling Problems, for advice on how to restart your periods). Do bear in mind, though, that just because you aren't menstruating doesn't mean you can't get pregnant. Remember, ovulation occurs before your period starts.

WHEN ARE YOU OVULATING?

If you aren't sure whether or not you are ovulating, there are a number of ways in which you can determine whether and when you are.

- Ovulation predictor kits are available from your chemist and offer a simple method of predicting ovulation just before it happens by detecting a subtle change in hormone levels. However, generally for women with PCOS and irregular periods they aren't reliable. (See Chapter Three, page 91, for more information and explanation on the above.)

- Checking cervical mucus. The mucus can be thick, white or pale yellow and sticky. As ovulation approaches the mucus becomes more copious, clear and elastic – a bit like egg white.

- Some women can tell when they are ovulating without any form of testing because they experience discomfort near the middle of their cycle for a day or so, just before the egg is released, along with symptoms such as breast tenderness, increased libido and a dull pain or ache in the ovary that is about to release an egg.

NFP is often recommended by preconceptual care advisers as a form of contraception, but it isn't foolproof. New research has even suggested that there could be no time in the month that it is safe to have sex. 'It may be the case that for a large proportion of the female population natural birth control is simply not an option,' says Dr Roger Pierson of the University of Saskatchewan, Canada, who led a study and whose findings were published in the medical journal Fertility and Sterility in July 2003. It also takes about four or five months to learn the method properly and become confident and comfortable with it, so if you really don't want to get pregnant right now it's not a good choice.

STEP THREE: DE-STRESS

'I'm a night nurse in a hospice and it's sometimes really hard to switch off from the pain, loneliness and suffering I see every day. Whenever I

feel really tired and anxious my symptoms get worse – especially the hair loss. I haven't had a regular period in years. I'm 30 next month and have been trying for a baby for two years. I went to my doctor to discuss my fertility and he told me that I might have to consider changing jobs, as the nature of the work I do and the fact that I work nights is stressful both emotionally and physically. You see stress may be making my symptoms worse and making it harder for me to get pregnant.' JENNY, 29

If you've got PCOS stress management is important. Recent research from the University of Birmingham and published in the online journal Genetics has suggested that the high testosterone levels associated with PCOS could be caused by a fault in the way the body processes the stress hormone cortisol. Cortisol, the active form of the hormone, can be turned into cortisone, the inactive form, by enzymes in the body. Researchers have found some women do not have these enzymes. This means that their bodies cannot process cortisol properly, which causes higher levels of testosterone to be produced.

So watching your stress levels is of great significance if you've got PCOS. Also if you want to get pregnant it's important too. Why? Because too much stress not only triggers PCOS symptoms it can also make them worse, including weight gain and irregular periods which, as we have seen, can both interfere with conception.

Dr Rosalind Bramwell of Liverpool University and Dr Robert Delman from the Roehamptom Institute, UK, believe that stress is both an emotional and a physical state that has very real effects on a human's hormonal system – in particular the output of sex hormones – due to its disturbance of the pituitary gland, which controls the process. It can also affect testosterone levels, interfering with ovulation and, of course, making symptoms of PCOS worse.

Stress and Your Periods

Prolonged disturbance to your menstrual cycle may not always be due to PCOS but could be due to the pressure you are under. It's not unusual to hear of women who have had problems trying to get pregnant for years, conceiving once the pressure is lifted. Studies show that extreme stress can stop ovulation.[49] For example, women going through bereavement or other kinds of trauma often stop having periods altogether. The women's hospital of the Berlin Charlottenburg in Germany found that out of approximately 2,000 couples being investigated for fertility in the late 1980s, in a quarter of all cases the cause was stress. It's not just extreme stress either – everyday episodes and experiences can all take their toll. For example, the prospect of a driving test can be enough to make you miss a period.

A recent study by Oxford University showed high stress levels can affect fertility directly. Researchers followed 274 healthy women aged 18–40 planning a pregnancy.

Markers for two stress hormones – adrenalin, the body's fight or flight hormone, and cortisol, connected with chronic stress – were measured in saliva. Women with the highest levels of alpha-amylase (an indicator of adrenalin levels) had about a 12% reduced chance of getting pregnant during their fertile days that month compared with those with the lowest levels of the marker. No difference in the chance of becoming pregnant was found with cortisol.

Dr Cecilia Pyper, of the National Perinatal Epidemiology Unit at the University of Oxford, said their study aimed to improve understanding of the factors that influence pregnancy in normal healthy women. 'This is the first study to find that a biological measure of stress is associated with a woman's chances of becoming pregnant that month,' she told the BBC. The findings support the idea that couples should aim to stay as relaxed as they can about trying for a baby. In some people's cases, it might be relevant to look at relaxation techniques, counselling and even approaches like yoga and meditation.'[50]

Stress and Fertility

Stress also hampers fertility because it produces unhealthy sperm and eggs, or both, and pregnancies created by damaged sperm or eggs usually result in early miscarriage.[51] What's more, higher than normal levels of stress hormone can also affect your libido because they can have a knock-on effect on the hormones – oestrogen and testosterone – that power sex drive. Not having enough sex or, as some experts believe, not enjoying sex if you do, is a prime cause of infertility.

Stress can affect male fertility too. It can influence a man's libido as well as his sperm. Research has shown that men under stress at work or home are more likely to have poor sperm quality and may experience poor fertility.[52]

Progressive fertility units such as the Beth Israel Hospital in Boston, USA, and the Harvard Behavioral Medicine Program have been including stress reduction in their programmes for 15 years. 'Our experience at the Division of Behavioral Medicine in the Beth Israel Deaconess Medical Center (and this is backed up by research) is that women with long-term infertility may well increase their chances of conception when they reduce their levels of stress and depression,' says Alice Domar, Director of the Mind/Body Institute at the centre.[53]

The International Europe survey of 2000 has identified stressful work as a major factor in infertility.[54] It seems that high public contact jobs, and high stress jobs such as air stewardess, teacher or nurse, increases the risk of miscarriage. Whatever the reason for your stress – be it anxiety about PCOS and/or your fertility, or exhaustion from too much exercise, or worries about your job, or upset because of troubles in your relationship – you may well find that this interferes with your health and fertility.

Stress is a fact of life so you can't avoid it but you can find ways to manage it. In fact, simply recognizing that you are stressed or anxious can be an important step.

Stress Management Tips

Healthy Eating

Any stress management regime needs to begin with a healthy eating plan (see Step Four below). Taking time to eat a balanced diet at regular mealtimes will ensure your body remains healthy and able to cope during stressful times.

Take Vitamins and Minerals

Take a multivitamin and mineral. It's your adrenal glands which produce the stress hormones – cortisol and adrenaline – and when you are under too much pressure they start to wear down and overproduce not just cortisol and adrenaline but testosterone too. Excess cortisol, adrenaline and testosterone will not only make PCOS worse but also drive your body towards irregular periods and subfertility. The adrenals rely on vitamins C, B5 and B6, zinc and magnesium and these are rapidly depleted when you are under stress, so a good multivitamin and mineral supplement every day makes sense.

Get Enough Sleep

Not getting enough quality sleep, which women with PCOS are prone to, makes it harder to handle stress and affects quality of life, according to a poll by the US National Sleep Foundation. In addition to raising stress hormones, research shows that sleep deprivation results in hormonal imbalance, therefore increasing the risk of infertility.[55] Amazingly enough, just one night of short sleep duration can induce insulin resistance, as it has such a profound effect on the body's glucose metabolism, says the latest research, published in The Endocrine Society's *Journal of Clinical Endocrinology & Metabolism* (JCEM).[56] And as we have seen, insulin resistance can contribute to hormonal imbalances in PCOS.[57] A good night's sleep is the best tonic you can have but it's important to realize that quality, not quantity, is the key. A recent study at Brigham and Women's Hospital in Boston, USA showed that a good night's sleep makes you feel happier and more relaxed, but those who had under six hours or over ten hours became irritable. Seven to eight hours seems ample for most people, but six hours of good quality sleep beats a restless nine hours.

To encourage a good night's sleep avoid eating, drinking or exercise at least two hours before you go to sleep. Try to stick to a regular bedtime, preferably before midnight, and a regular waking time. Keep fresh air circulating in your bedroom; the brain's sleep centre works better with oxygen. Make sure your bedroom isn't too noisy, light, untidy, hot or cold. A warm bath, perhaps with a few drops of lavender or neroli oil, can have a sedative quality. In fact, recent research has shown lavender essential oil can alter blood chemistry to relieve stress and therefore promote relaxation.[58] Simple relaxation techniques before you go to sleep, such as gentle stretching or meditation, can also help.

Meditate
Meditation is a great way to lower both physical and mental stress. To try meditation by yourself, find a quiet place where you won't be interrupted. Make sure you are comfortable, and then start to imagine each part of your body from your toes to your scalp relaxing, while mentally repeating a neutral thought (try a colour). When other thoughts break through the

calm just let them come and go. After 10 minutes open your eyes and sit quietly for a few moments before getting up.

Transcendental Meditation

Why not try transcendental meditation, which is thought to be up to eight times more beneficial to your health than other relaxation techniques. Tuition consists of a one-hour session where you are given a mantra to repeat over and over as you sit quietly. Follow-up classes fine-tune your technique. You must then meditate for 20 minutes twice a day and the proven benefits include increased mental and physical alertness and better coping skills when under stress.

Massage

Massage can help. The sense of wellbeing you get from a massage can lower the amount of stress hormones, such as cortisol, circulating throughout your body. Either book a session with a qualified practitioner, or if you have time and think it would be fun, use a good book or a video to learn some simple techniques for yourself.

Yoga

Take up Yoga. MIND, the UK's leading mental health charity, recommends Yoga as the single most effective stress buster. Yoga has been around for thousands of years, and although its many famous fans have helped it become cool now, its benefits remain constant. The poses aim to bring your mind, body and breathing together to improve posture and physical health and bring a sense of calm. One study from Boston University School of Medicine (BUSM) found that yoga may be superior to other forms of exercise in its positive effect on lifting mood and relieving anxiety due to its effect on releasing chemicals in the brain.[59]

Avoid Triggers

Think about how you react to stress and identify those people and situations that trigger it. You can't avoid every trigger but you don't have to invite them into your life.

Relaxation Techniques

Use simple relaxation techniques to deal with short-term stress. For example, if you get tense when stuck in traffic, try simple techniques such as tensing your muscles hard and relaxing them, or deep breathing for a count of 10, or daydreaming about a holiday. Other techniques include drinking calming herbal teas like chamomile, having a good laugh, chatting to a friend, reading a good book or listening to soothing music. Set aside 10 or 20 minutes a day to relax, no matter what.

Exercise

The exercise you're doing in this preconceptual care stage is also great for beating stress. Not only does it stimulate the body's pituitary gland to release tension and give you a natural high, it also tires you out so you sleep better no matter how much your brain is racing. Research also shows that regular exercise makes you less tense and better able to cope with stress.

Forget Perfection

Try not to be a perfectionist. Let the dishes sit in the dishwasher a little longer, return that call tomorrow, wear clothes you feel comfortable in.

Learn to manage your time more effectively and each day won't seem such a struggle. Plan your day and prioritize what needs to be done. Tackle one task at a time and allow extra time for the unexpected.

Breathe Deeply
Stress forces you to take shallow breaths which don't let your body get rid of tension the way a deep breath can. A large lung full of air centres and calms you. Most of us take tiny breaths. Practise this breathing technique the next time you feel stressed: to a count of four breathe in through your nose, right down into your stomach, hold for one, then push the breath out again for a count of four.

Share Your Problems
Simply talking to friends, family and partners can ease stress. If you don't feel that you have anyone you can talk to, a trained counsellor can help you get in touch with your feelings and give you tips on stress management. You may also find that you get a great deal of support and encouragement from other women with PCOS. If you haven't already, think about joining a PCOS support group – you'll find contact details in the Resource Guide. Finally, don't forget that your very best friend and support is you. Instead of being your own worst enemy, be as nice to yourself as you are to your friends.

STEP FOUR: EAT FRESH, HEALTHY FOOD, PACKED WITH FERTILITY-BOOSTING NUTRIENTS

> 'My mum started seeing a nutritionist when her weight spiraled out of control and to give her support I went to the meetings with her. To encourage her I also cut down on saturated fat and sugar, increased my fruit and vegetable intake, and most important of all started eating

breakfast and snacking regularly on healthy nibbles during the day, so that I wouldn't have a massive chocolate binge on the way home from work. I also started taking a multivitamin and mineral. As if by magic my periods – after being irregular for years – now appear every 28 or so days. In the next year or so I want to start thinking of babies and it's good to know that with regular periods and a healthy diet I stand a very good chance of getting pregnant.' FRANCESCA, 29

You really can improve your fertility by what you eat, says Dr Margaret Rayman, Director of the MSC Course in Nutrition Medicine at the University of Surrey. The food you eat affects every single cell and system in your entire body and is needed to produce healthy eggs (and sperm) for the development of your baby when you get pregnant. A healthy, balanced diet in the preconception period will not only boost your chances of having a healthy baby, it will also help keep your weight down and your blood sugar levels in balance. If your blood sugars are not balanced then your hormones, which control your fertility, will not work properly either.

Balancing Blood Sugar Levels

The link between blood sugar levels and hormone balance was first recognized by Dr Katharina Dalton when she realized that her patients who suffered from PMS found their symptoms were relieved by eating regularly. The 'little and often' approach to eating prevents blood sugar levels from dropping and stops adrenaline being released. Adrenaline blocks the utilization of progesterone in the second half of the menstrual cycle and this was causing symptoms of PMS. The answer was to stabilize blood sugar levels by getting patients to eat properly so that adrenaline didn't interfere with their hormone balance. Dalton's work has huge implications for fertility. If progesterone is blocked it reduces the chances of conception since this hormone is needed to maintain the womb lining at the start of a pregnancy.

There is also a clear link between blood sugar balance problems and conditions such as PCOS, diabetes, poor eating habits and excess weight. If your blood sugar levels zoom up and down chaotically, not only will this affect your hormones but it can also spark off sugar cravings, food obsessions and poor eating habits, which in turn can lead to weight gain.

Healthy eating can restore your blood sugar and hormone balance, improve your energy levels, and help you lose weight as well as addressing irregular periods and subfertility. 'Eating a healthy, well-balanced diet of fresh, whole foods in combination with moderate exercise is,' in the words of Helen Mason, Senior Lecturer in Reproductive Endocrinology at St George's Hospital Medical School, London, 'the first line of treatment for PCOS infertility patients.'

Your Healthy PCOS Diet

But what is a healthy diet for PCOS? It follows basic rules – sufficient complex carbohydrate, moderate amounts of protein, sufficient essential fats, a minimum of saturated fats and lots of water.

Water
Water is an essential but often forgotten ingredient in a healthy eating plan. Water intake is vital for hormonal function and you need to drink lots to keep your hormonal systems at their best. Try to drink at least one and a half litres or two and three-quarter pints, or six to eight glasses of fresh water a day.

Carbohydrates
To optimize your fertility you should eat plenty of unrefined complex

carbohydrates, which don't lead to a sudden rise in your blood sugar levels. This means choosing brown wholemeal grains, bread and pasta, instead of the refined white versions, which have been stripped of their valuable fibre content, and at least five portions of vegetables each day. Simple carbohydrates in the form of sweets, cakes and white sugar can all produce a sudden rise in blood sugar so it's important to avoid them.

Fruits are the exception here as they are a simple sugar and they are packed with fertility-boosting nutrients. You shouldn't cut fruit out but make sure you eat it with proteins, such as a few nuts or seeds, or some low-fat yogurt, which can slow down the effect on blood sugar.

We need fibre to keep our bowels healthy but it is also vital for our fertility because it can help keep our reproductive systems in optimum condition by helping clear out toxins and old hormone residues. It isn't difficult to increase your fibre intake. You don't need to add bran to everything, just eat more complex carbohydrates: wholegrain rice, bread and pasta, and plenty of fruits, vegetables, beans, nuts and seeds. Or choose lower GI fruits such as cherries, plums, peaches, grapefruits, apples, pears, dried apricots, oranges, strawberries and prunes.[60]

Protein
Protein is important for your fertility because it helps maintain blood sugar balance and gives your body the even supply of amino acids it needs to build and repair cells and manufacture hormones. Since your body can't store protein the way it does carbohydrate and fat, you need a constant supply and should aim to eat some high quality protein with every meal. Good sources of protein include low-fat dairy products, lean meat, eggs, pulses, beans, nuts and seeds.

Fats
Unfortunately fat in general has got a bad name, although it's the

saturated fats, found in animal meat and full-fat dairy products, that are harmful. Essential fatty acids (EFA), found in nuts, seeds and oily fish, play a crucial role in fertility and the development of a healthy baby.[61,62] Scientists have looked at their role in pregnancy and found they are crucial for the brain, eyes, and nervous system development of a growing baby. If you don't eat enough EFA, hormone production will also be compromised. It takes three months to build up your body's stores, so make sure that you eat some every day. Good sources include evening primrose oil, flaxseed oil, and oily fish. Have a handful of nuts every day or use a salad dressing made with a good quality nut or seed oil. The recommended daily dose is 1,000mg flaxseed oil.[d]

Pro-Fertility Vitamins and Minerals

A healthy balanced diet should ensure an adequate intake of every nutrient but some nutrients are more essential for your fertility than others:

VITAMIN E Infertile couples given vitamin E (200 IU per day for the female and 100 IU per day for the male), showed a significant increase in fertility in a preliminary human trial.[63] Vitamin E's beneficial role in female reproductive health has since been backed up by more recent research.[64] Food sources include wheatgerm, avocados, eggs, butter, wholemeal cereals, seeds, nuts, oily fish, broccoli. The recommended daily dose is 300–400 IU.

IRON Iron deficiency should always be checked during infertility investigation, as taking iron is known to have helped women regain their fertility.[65] Even a subtle deficiency could contribute to infertility in women.[66] Iron supplements given together with vitamin C (which increases the absorption of iron) have resulted in a number of women with fertility problems becoming pregnant, including one woman who had undergone nine years of unsuccessful fertility treatment.[67,68] Your requirement for iron increases once you get pregnant. It's always better to get iron from food sources than from a supplement because of the risk of constipation and heartburn. Food sources include eggs, fish, dried milk, dark green vegetables, lean red meat and pulses.

ZINC A zinc deficiency in women can lead to reduced fertility and increased risk of miscarriage.[69] It is vital for the development of unborn babies. Food sources include seafood, milk, whole grains and dried fruit. Oysters are an especially good source of Zinc. The recommended daily dose is 30 mg. New research published in 2010 from Northwestern University, USA, reveals healthy eggs need a tremendous amount of zinc to reach maturity and be ready for fertilization – a finding that may ultimately help physicians assess the best eggs for fertility treatment. In a study with mice, scientists discovered the egg becomes ravenous for zinc and acquires a 50% increase in the metal in order to reach full maturity before becoming fertilized. The flood of zinc appears to flip a switch so the egg can progress through the final stages of meiosis. Meiosis is when the egg sheds all but one copy of its maternal chromosomes before it can be fertilized by a sperm and become an embryo.

Northwestern scientists also used small molecules to block the accumulation of zinc by the maturing egg. They found an insufficient accumulation of zinc caused all the eggs to pause prematurely at the beginning stage of meiosis. The progression of meiosis was restored by returning zinc to the eggs.[70]

MANGANESE Research has shown that women with low manganese levels are more likely to give birth to a baby with a malformation.[71] Food sources include tea, nuts, wholegrains and legumes. The recommended daily dose is 5 mg.

PABA   Some previously infertile women have become pregnant after supplementing with 100 mg PABA (para-aminobenzoic acid), four times per day.[72] PABA is believed to increase the ability of oestrogen to facilitate fertility.

B VITAMINS   Another important vitamin for your fertility is vitamin B12 (found in sardines, eggs, spirulina and seaweed) according to a recent study.[73] Research has also shown that giving vitamin B6 (good sources are avocados, lentils, and watermelon) to women who have trouble conceiving increases their fertility. In one study, 12 out of 14 women who had been trying to conceive succeeded after taking vitamin B6 daily for six months.[74] The recommended daily dose of each is 50 mg.

FOLIC ACID   Until recently this was just another B vitamin, but now conclusive research has shown its vital role in preventing spina bifida. Food sources include green beans, spinach, brussel sprouts, milk and fruit. This is such an important nutrient that all doctors recommend taking it as a supplement in the preconception period. The recommended daily dose is 400 mcg.

VITAMIN C   Vitamin C may also play a role. Research in the seventies showed that when given to women undergoing fertility treatment it can help trigger ovulation, and recent research is confirming Vitamin C's crucial role.[75] Vitamin C is found in raw fruits and vegetables, especially citrus fruits, blackcurrants, kiwi fruit, mangoes, red peppers, strawberries, green sprouting vegetables like brussel sprouts, water cress and parsley. The recommended daily dose is 40 mg.

Vitamin C, along with vitamin E, may also play a role in preserving your fertility for longer. An interesting study was conducted at the Department of Pediatrics, Obstetrics and Gynecology, Faculty of Medicine, University of Valencia, Spain.[76] It aimed to ascertain whether dietary supplementation with a mixture of vitamins C and E could prevent the maternal age-associated decrease in egg quality in mice. The study showed promising results, with the age-related reduction in ovulation rate partially prevented by high doses of these vitamins. Studies have yet to be done on humans but these findings may have direct implications for preventing or delaying maternal age-associated infertility in humans.

L-ARGININE   Supplementation with the amino acid L-arginine has been shown to improve fertilization rates in women with a previous history of failed attempts at in vitro (test tube) fertilization.[77]

VITAMIN A   It is also important to have good levels of vitamin A at the point of conception because it is essential to the developing embryo, and in studies with animals a deficiency of vitamin A produced newborns with birth defects. High doses of vitamin A are not advised as this can also cause birth defects, but it seems that vegetable sources of beta carotene, which your body can turn into vitamin A, are safe.[78,79] Vitamin A (beta carotene) is found in carrots, tomatoes, mangos, pumpkins, cabbage, spinach, and broccoli. The recommended daily dose is up to 500 IU.

SELENIUM   In women, selenium deficiency is linked to miscarriage. Food sources include herring, tuna, whole wheat, broccoli and garlic. The recommended daily dose is 100 mcg.

MAGNESIUM   According to research in the late seventies and again in the nineties, magnesium is one of the most important minerals affecting a woman's ability to conceive and the maintenance of the pregnancy itself.[80] Food sources include dairy products, nuts, vegetables, meat, cooked brown rice and sunflower seeds. The recommended daily dose is 300 mg.

For Him

Your partner needs to ensure that he eats a wide range of nutrients too. Research has shown that the following nutrients are of special importance to men because of their impact on sperm quality and quantity: vitamin A, B complex, magnesium, zinc, calcium, selenium, vitamin E, folic acid and manganese. Plus, omega-3 fatty acids that the body makes from foods such as oily fish and soybean oil, may help boost the sperm count, and motility in men with poor sperm quality, says a recent University of Illinois study. More research is needed, but early indications suggest that docosahexaenoic acid (DHA) is important for healthy sperm.[81]

Combine a nutrient-rich diet with daily sex (or ejaculating daily) for seven days and you can improve men's sperm quality by reducing the amount of DNA damage, according to an Australian study presented to the 25th annual meeting of the European Society of Human Reproduction and Embryology in Amsterdam.[82]

Taking Supplements

Many nutrients important for fertility are quite fragile and easily destroyed by heating, cooking and storage, so as a rule of thumb try to eat your food as fresh and as close to its natural state – preferably organic – as possible. Avoid food that is processed and packed with chemicals, additives and preservatives. Taking a good quality daily multivitamin and mineral is also a good idea.

Women who take daily multivitamin tablets can double their chances of getting pregnant say researchers from the University of Leeds. Researchers believe that taking a daily multivitamin can help produce better quality eggs.[83] A study presented to the European Society of Human Reproduction and Embryology in July 2001 showed that in 215 women in Leeds, UK, undergoing IVF and taking the vitamin pill, the fluid surrounding the eggs was enriched with vitamin C and E, which the researchers believe can give the egg a crucial boost. Leader of the research, gynaecology senior registrar Dr Sara Matthews, said: 'My theory is that it might apply to anyone trying for pregnancy.'

Supplements can be effective in rebalancing your hormones and improving health and fertility, but since all nutrients depend on each other to function properly, it is important to take a good multivitamin and mineral as the basic foundation and then add in other individual nutrients on top to meet the required daily dose.

It's also important to remember that supplements are no substitute for a healthy diet. Dr Ann Walker, a medical herbalist and nutrition research scientist based at the University of Reading's Hugh Sinclair Unit of Human Nutrition for many years says, 'There is no point in any medication or supplement coming in to correct symptoms that are caused by a bad diet and unhealthy lifestyle. It is important to get the diet and lifestyle healthy first and then treat any outstanding health issues.'

Before you go to the health food shop to buy supplements it might be a good idea to see a dietician or nutritionist, preferably one with an interest in fertility and, in an ideal world, with experience of PCOS patients. It pays to get a health professional to give you advice about diet and lifestyle and check, using blood, sweat or muscle-testing, what you personally might be short of, rather than buying a general prepregnancy or health-boosting formula which may not actually help you that much.

Your Fertility Eating Plan

The fertility buffet (below) was created by Vicky Chudleigh, State Registered Dietician from Addenbrookes Hospital in Cambridge, UK, to show that eating well needn't be boring — and we've used that attitude to create the seven-day menu plan that follows for you.

A Week of PCOS Fertility-Boosting Menus

You can drink unlimited herbal teas and pure water throughout these days.

DAY ONE

Breakfast: poached egg on wholemeal toast; glass of freshly pressed apple juice

Mid-morning snack: pear and six almonds

Lunch: grilled chicken breast, small jacket potato, big mixed rainbow salad with red peppers, carrots, red onions, spinach and lettuce; sprinkled with sunflower seeds and flax seeds

Mid-afternoon snack: small bar organic dark chocolate and glass of skimmed organic milk or diluted fruit juice

Dinner: tofu or salmon, onion, pepper and broccoli kebabs on brown basmati rice, with green salad leaves; stewed dried apricots with a splash of yoghurt

DAY TWO

Breakfast: porridge made with skimmed or soya milk, sprinkled with chopped brazil nuts, dried apricots and dried figs; glass of freshly pressed apple juice

Mid-morning: large slice melon, handful of mixed seeds with raisins

Lunch: cheese or prawn salad platter with wholemeal pitta bread; fruit crumble with low-fat ice cream
Mid-afternoon: glass of almond or cashew nut milk and crackers
Dinner: mixed seafood or tofu paella with green salad; fresh fruit salad

DAY THREE

Breakfast: muesli or granola with extra flax seeds and wheatgerm sprinkled on it; glass of freshly pressed pineapple juice
Mid-morning: glass of skimmed organic or soya milk and an apple
Lunch: three-bean chilli tomato casserole with small jacket potato or wholegrain rice; onion and mint salad
Mid-afternoon: handful of dried apricots or figs with five brazil nuts
Dinner: seafood, chicken or vegetarian sausage pizza – made with wholemeal pizza bases; piled high with freshly cut vegetables and tomato sauce; green salad; sliced mango with lime juice

DAY FOUR

Breakfast: bowl of mixed berries with chopped nuts, flax seeds and low-fat yoghurt topping; glass of freshly pressed pear juice
Mid-morning: apple and sunflower seeds
Lunch: mozzarella, avocado and tomato salad with lemon juice and hempseed oil dressing; wholegrain bread roll; fruit salad
Mid-afternoon: glass of skimmed milk or diluted fruit juice and wholemeal fruit scone
Dinner: chicken or tofu stir fry with garlic, ginger, soy sauce and lots of crunchy vegetables – carrots, broccoli; onions, peppers, green beans, baby corn, plus wholegrain rice; small bar dark chocolate

DAY FIVE

Breakfast: lean bacon or tofu sausages and scrambled eggs; glass freshly pressed apple juice

Mid-morning: Twiglets or low-fat pretzel snack

Lunch: bowl of mixed vegetable soup sprinkled with flax and pumpkin seeds; tuna or hummus sandwich on wholegrain bread

Mid-afternoon: apple, three dried apricots and three walnuts

Dinner: lentil dahl with wholegrain rice or chapattis; green salad; fresh pineapple

DAY SIX

Breakfast: boiled egg with wholegrain toast soldiers; freshly pressed apple juice

Mid-morning: glass of skimmed or soya milk and five brazil nuts

Lunch: fish pie (topped with mashed potato, not pastry); mixed rainbow salad

Mid-afternoon: two Jaffa cakes; apple

Dinner: fragrant thai green or red curry – choose fish, chicken or bean curd – with brown basmati rice; mixed fruit salad with chopped nuts, seeds and yoghurt topping

DAY SEVEN

Breakfast: wholemeal toasted muffin with lean bacon or tofu sausage and ketchup; glass of freshly pressed apple juice

Mid-morning: small bunch of grapes and handful mixed nuts

Lunch: grilled fish, chicken breast, or quorn fillet, with roasted mixed vegetables (peppers, onions, sweet potato, carrots, courgettes and asparagus, in a tray, drizzled with olive oil and lots of crushed garlic, roasted until tender)

Mid-afternoon: glass of skimmed organic or nut milk and one small cookie

Dinner: luxury mixed salad with leaves, crispy vegetable chunks (onion, peppers, carrots, sweet peas), cheese cubes, cashew nuts, beetroot, sliced eggs, with hot garlic baguette; dark chocolate mousse with raspberries

The Fertility Buffet

Blinis topped with smoked salmon and horseradish
Crostinis topped with pesto and roasted red peppers
Sunflower, pumpkin, sesame seed and brazil nut bread
Extra virgin oil with Parmesan for dipping

PLATTERS
A selection of cold and cured meats
A selection of fish goujons, mini crab cakes and sweet chilli dip and
   calamari
Goats cheese, thyme and tomato tart

SALADS
Cucumber, fennel, celery and chicory salad
A pasta salad with shredded watercress baby spinach and pesto
Sliced beef tomatoes with a basil dressing

DESSERTS *Fruit Kebabs*
Dacquoise, a delicate combination of almond meringue with cream
   and an apricot coulis
Rich chocolate mousse
A selection of European cheeses and biscuits
Chocolate brazil nuts

The sunflower, pumpkin and sesame seed bread contains vitamin E, which is claimed to be an aphrodisiac because of its effects on boosting circulation. It is also an antioxidant and needed for fertility. Brazil nuts and mini crab cakes are both excellent sources of selenium and required for sperm motility. Selenium also minimizes the risk of miscarriages. All the other items on the menu were selected for their fertility-boosting qualities. For example, spinach, together with dark green leafy vegetables, provides the folate required to reduce the risk of neural tube defect in the developing baby. Cheese contains calcium, zinc and vitamin A, which are all needed for healthy reproduction and libido.

STEP FIVE: DETOX YOUR LIFESTYLE

There are many things in our day-to-day lives that can make symptoms of PCOS worse, and anything that makes irregular periods worse will, of course, make it harder for you to get pregnant. There are now over 300 chemicals that didn't exist 50 years ago, that can collect in your body, rob you of nutrients and interfere with hormonal health.[84]

Every day a sea of hormone-disturbing toxins surrounds us. They are in cigarette smoke; in pesticides and herbicides in our soil; in chemicals and additives in the food we eat; contaminants in the water we drink; environmental chemicals in solvents, plastics and adhesives; as well as all the toxins we absorb through the skin in make-up, hair dyes and household cleaning products. Our bodies don't need or want any of these chemicals and have to work hard to process (metabolize) them and get rid of (detoxify) them, through the liver, kidneys, lymph and digestive system. In the process of metabolizing and detoxing, our bodies also lose vital nutrients – nutrients we need to feel healthy, beat symptoms of PCOS and boost fertility.

These toxins have also been linked to birth defects and hormonal disruption so great, that some of them are now called GED or general endocrine disrupters. They could be interfering with your ability to conceive because of the damage they cause to your ovulation cycle and possibly your eggs, as well as to a man's sperm production. 'The cause of many infertility cases (up to 20 percent) remains unexplained,' says Dr John Sussman, Fellow of the American College of Obstetricians and Gynecology and founder of the 'Preparation for Pregnancy' programme at the New Milford Hospital, Connecticut. 'Some think low-level exposure to toxins may eventually be found to be the culprit.'

It's not all doom and gloom though – you can detox your lifestyle in simple ways to promote hormonal balance and fertility.

Keep Your Liver, Kidneys and Lymph Happy!

These organs are your body's own powerhouse of detoxing and by keeping them healthy you can help your body flush out harmful toxins and process old hormones to stop them causing imbalances (for more on liver protection see page 107 in Chapter Three). Keep your kidneys happy by drinking lots of pure water, balancing your protein intake with low GI carbs (that cause a gradual, less pronounced rise in blood sugar) and keep your lymph system in good order with regular self-massage and exercise.

Smoking

Fertility experts agree that cigarettes and alcohol can be damaging. The advice to you and your partner is to give up, or at the very least cut down.

Over 600 chemicals are allowed into cigarettes, revealed a UK Report published in 2000 by the then Health Secretary Alan Milburn. Smoking is a significant antinutrient and it reduces the level of vitamin C in the bloodstream. Smokers also have high levels of cadmium, a heavy toxic metal that can stop the utilization of zinc needed for a healthy menstrual cycle.

Scientists at Massachusetts General Hospital in Boston have found that smoking can trigger infertility in both men and women.[85] Other studies confirm that women who do not smoke are twice as likely to get pregnant as women who do smoke.[86] Cigarettes reduce oestrogen levels, and lowered oestrogen levels cut down the number of fertile years a woman has left to conceive, cause irregular periods, and make eggs and cervical mucus less hospitable to sperm. In short, the more you smoke, the less likely you are to conceive.[87] In fact, women whose mothers smoked during their pregnancy are less likely to conceive compared with those whose mothers were nonsmokers.[88] So strong is the evidence against smoking that, although there isn't an official anti-smoking policy from the Human Fertilization and Embryology Authority (HFEA), they strongly advise against it when anybody is undergoing fertility treatment. Many countries and US states now ban smoking in public places because of its detrimental effect on health. And countries including New Zealand and Wales make being a non-smoker an essential for any couples seeking IVF treatment, with many individual clinics also making this a pre-requisite of treatment.

Smoking damages almost all aspects of sexual, reproductive and child health, according to the British Medical Association (BMA). It is one of the major causes of impotence in men, is responsible for up to 5,000 miscarriages a year, reduces the chances of successful IVF and is implicated in cases of cervical cancer. Recent research shows smoking adds the equivalent of 10 years to the reproductive age of a

20-year-old woman seeking to have a baby by in vitro fertilisation and has a 'devastating' impact on a couple's chances of a successful delivery, according to scientists from the Netherlands.[89] Dutch researchers found smoking reduced the technique's success rate by about 30 percent and increased the risk of miscarriage by almost a quarter in a study into the success rate of first-cycle IVF treatment in more than 8,000 women. And it's not only women smoking – men who smoke reduce the chances of successful IVF too, and the negative effect increases as they get older.[90,91]

It says smoking reduces the chances of a woman conceiving by up to 40 percent per cycle. Also, women who smoke during pregnancy are three times more likely to have a low birth-weight baby. There is also evidence that smoking may increase the risk of certain fetal malformations, such as cleft lip and palate. Women who smoke have also been found to produce smaller volumes of lower quality breast milk. Passive smoking is linked to cot death (sudden infant death symdrome), premature birth, respiratory infection in children and the development of childhood asthma.

Dr Vivienne Nathanson, the BMA's Head of Science and Ethics, said: 'The sheer scale of damage that smoking causes to reproductive and child health is shocking. Women are generally aware that they should not smoke while pregnant but the message needs to be far stronger. Men and women who think they might want children one day should bin cigarettes. And we're not just talking about having children. Men who want to continue to enjoy sex should forget about lighting up, given the strong evidence that smoking is a major cause of male sexual impotence.'

Deborah Arnott, Director of the anti smoking charity ASH, said: 'The BMA report clearly shows the devastating impact of smoking on generations to come. Stopping smoking should be the number one priority for anyone who wants to have children. This is important not just to increase the chances of conception but also to give your child the best start in life.'

Alcohol

Alcohol can also interfere with hormonal health. Research has shown that women who drink heavily stop ovulating and menstruating and take longer to conceive. A study in the *British Medical Journal* in 1998 states categorically that women should avoid alcohol when trying to conceive. Alcohol may prevent enough progesterone being produced by the egg capsule, and progesterone is one of the major players in ensuring a pregnancy stays put. Even moderate drinking is linked to an increased risk of infertility in some women.[92] In one preliminary study, there was a greater than 50 percent reduction in the probability of conception in a menstrual cycle during which participants consumed alcohol.

We would suggest that, if you have PCOS and are trying to bring your symptoms under control and boost your fertility, you only drink alcohol in moderation (say, one glass of wine, spirits or beer a day). Any more than that could have a harmful effect on your fertility. There are many lower alcohol wines and spirits available today and an increasing number of organic options.

It's not just you who needs to cut down, your partner does too. A man can wipe out his sperm count for up to three months after a single heavy drinking session, according to Anthony Harsh, andrologist at Whipps Cross Hospital, UK. This is because alcohol reduces the level of vital sperm-making hormones, and preconceptual care experts often insist that a man who wants to father a healthy child should stop drinking for at least three months before trying to get his partner pregnant.

Caffeine

You might also want to think about cutting down on the amount of caffeine in your diet. Drinking one to one and a half cups of coffee per day in one study, and about three or four cups per day in other studies, has been associated with delayed conception in women trying to get pregnant.[93-95] In another study, women who drank more than one cup of coffee per day had a 50 percent reduction in fertility, compared with women who drank less coffee.[96] Until recently, it was unclear why caffeine had this effect. But research published in the *British Journal of Pharmacology* in 2011 revealed that caffeine reduces muscle activity in the fallopian tubes that carry eggs from the ovaries to the womb. 'Our experiments were conducted in mice, but this finding goes a long way towards explaining why drinking caffeinated drinks can reduce a woman's chance of becoming pregnant,' says Professor Sean Ward from the University of Nevada School of Medicine, Reno.[97] In another, drinking three cups of decaffeinated coffee per day was associated with an increased risk of spontaneous abortion, and other research suggests that caffeine consumption compounded the negative effects of alcohol consumption on female fertility.[98-100, e]

Caffeine is found in regular coffee, black tea, green tea, some soft drinks, chocolate and many over-the-counter pharmaceuticals. While not every study finds that caffeine reduces female fertility, and the US National Institutes of Health and the American Heart Association suggest that drinking two cups of tea a day can reduce the risk of heart disease, many doctors recommend that women trying to get pregnant avoid caffeine or cut down.[101] So, overall it seems that, although you don't need to cut out coffee, tea, chocolate and colas altogether, you do need to cut down to no more than one or two cups a day or switch to herbal or fruit teas.

Medications

Medications that you or your partner may take can also interfere with your fertility and it is important that you are aware of their effects. When in doubt, if you need to take any kind of prescription drugs, have a chat with your doctor about its impact on your fertility. It is thought that commonly prescribed painkillers, such as ibuprofen, ketoprofen and naproxen, may increase the risk of miscarriage. 'Until we know more, these drugs should be avoided,' says Professor James Driffe from the Royal College of Obstetricians and Gynaecologists in London. Research gets updated all the time, so ask your GP about this.

Doubts have also been cast over the safety of paracetamol. Low-dose aspirin, however, seems to be an exception, according to a 2001 study at the Institute of Health Sciences in Oxford, and may actually have a beneficial effect, but this area hasn't been studied widely and further studies are needed to confirm the findings. The Royal College of Obstetrics and Gynaecology still advises women concerned about their fertility to check with their doctor first before taking aspirin, paracetamol or any kind of painkiller.

Detox Your Food

If you have PCOS and are concerned about your fertility, it really is important to make sure that what ends up on your plate is as fresh and as nutritious as possible. You need all the nutrients you can get to beat your symptoms and boost your fertility, and that means avoiding food that has been chemically treated.

Chemicals, pesticides and preservatives used on food to keep them pest-free or make them last longer, taste different or look different, can build up over time.[102] Xenoestrogens or synthetic oestrogens are environmental toxins derived from pesticides and plastics. We eat them in our food, drink them in our water and store them in our body fat and they can have a negative effect on our hormones.

We highly recommend that you and your partner eat organic food, wherever possible. Organic food often contains higher levels of nutrients and is free from chemical pesticides, herbicides and artificial fertilizers. To cut the cost of going organic you could either join an organic food box scheme, where fruits and vegetables are delivered to your door from local producers, or you could visit your local farmers' market to get a better deal. If going organic isn't practical for you, there are ways you can protect yourself against xenoestrogens:

- If you can't go completely organic, eat just organic fruits and vegetables at least always wash all fruits and vegetables thoroughly.

- Drink at least six glasses of water a day – add fruit juice if this gets boring – and filter your water. Use a stainless steel filtration system fitted under your sink, if possible, not a plastic one. Alternatively use a water filter.

- Reduce your intake of fatty animal products (meat and dairy) as xenoestrogens accumulate in fat.

- Never heat food in plastic containers and don't wrap food in plastic – the plastic contains toxins that can be absorbed in your food.

- Think brown – go for unrefined complex carbohydrates (brown rice, wholemeal pasta, brown bread). Avoid white bread, pasta, biscuits, cakes and refined foods.

- Eat a leafy, green vegetable a day. Cruciferous vegetables such as broccoli, cauliflower or cabbage can boost the liver's ability to detoxify harmful chemicals.

Detoxing Your Life

At home and at work we are all exposed to toxins and health risks that could pose a threat to our fertility. For example, research shows that women who are exposed to heavy metals and chemicals, such as lead, aluminium and cadmium, often have problems with their menstrual cycle, experiencing hormone imbalances and miscarriages and taking longer to get pregnant.[103]

BPA, fertility and PCOS – the lowdown

There is increasing discussion among reproductive experts and nutritionists, about the role that modern chemicals play in our fertility. And recent research suggests reducing exposure to a chemical called bisphenol A (BPA) could be a sensible precaution. At the time of writing, more research needs to be done, as the current evidence remains controversial, as some experts believe it is not robust enough to reflect the real levels of BPA that we are exposed to in daily life. This is because doses used on animals in a laboratory setting are far greater than those in an everyday environment. However several studies now link this chemical to fertility issues in women with PCOS, in men, and in pregnancy.[104–106] A recent World Health Organization conference on the issue says more research is needed on the effects of lower doses on humans. And as research evolves, a new study has revealed BPA collects in human tissues at much faster rates than previously thought, through diet.[107]

A recent study from the University of Athens Medical School in Greece, has discovered that women with PCOS may be more vulnerable to BPA, which is used to make clear, shatterproof plastic, and found in items as diverse as water bottles, dental fillings, glasses lenses, CDs and DVDs, thermal paper coating receipts and tickets; and epoxy resins coating the inside of food and beverage cans. Blood levels of BPA were 60 percent higher in lean women with PCOS and 30 percent higher in obese women with PCOS, than in the healthy female group. Additionally, as BPA levels increased, so did concentrations of the male sex hormone testosterone. 'Excessive secretion of male hormones, as seen in PCOS, interfere with BPA detoxification by the liver, leading to accumulation of blood levels of BPA,' said Professor Evanthia Diamanti-Kandarakis, study co-author. 'BPA also affects androgen metabolism, creating a vicious circle between androgens and BPA.'[104] In another study, from Argentina, rats exposed to very high levels of BPA early in life (several thousand times higher than levels humans are thought to be exposed to) developed symptoms resembling those of women with PCOS, including reduced ovulation, elevated testosterone and irregularities in the secretion of GnRH, a hormone in the brain that normally regulates the activity of other reproductive hormones.[105]

A small-scale University of California, San Francisco-led study has identified the first evidence in humans that exposure to BPA may compromise the quality of a woman's eggs retrieved for IVF. As blood levels of BPA in the women studied doubled, the percentage of eggs that fertilized normally declined by 50 percent, according to the research team.[108]

Parental exposure to BPA during pregnancy is currently being investigated due to possible links with decreased birth weight of offspring, compared with offspring from families without parental BPA exposure in the workplace; and also links with potential neurological changes in babies.

In men, increased exposure to BPA has been found to lower testosterone levels, reduce sexual function, and decrease sperm concentration, total sperm count, sperm vitality and sperm motility.[109-113]

Take action – plastic protection

'If you have PCOS, you should be alert to the potential risks and take care of yourself by avoiding excessive everyday consumption of food or drink from plastic containers,' says Professor Diamanti-Kandarakis. Women's health expert and nutritionist Marilyn Glenville (www.marilynglenville.com), offers this practical advice:

- Buy drinks in glass bottles.
- If you do use plastic bottles, change them regularly – if they get damaged it can increase the likelihood of chemicals leaching into the water. And don't leave them in strong sunlight as higher temperatures increase the likelihood that chemicals leach into the water.
- Avoid using harsh detergents or very hot liquids in plastic water bottles, baby bottles or plastic containers – set them on a low temperature wash if you use the dishwasher.
- Reduce your use of canned foods.
- Avoid microwaving food in plastic containers.
- Wash your hands regularly if you often handle thermal paper such as airline tickets, event and cinema tickets, labels and receipts.
- Use plastic wraps and cookware made of polyethylene that doesn't contain plasticisers. If the product doesn't make this clear, don't buy it.
- Don't store fatty food in plastic wrap, as the chemicals leach into the fat. If you buy hard cheese wrapped in plastic use a knife to shave off the surface layer.

Lead

Lead is a heavy, toxic metal that is naturally present in the earth, but we get exposure to it from lead pipes. Lead has been used in the past to induce abortion, and women who live in lead-polluted areas have a higher level of miscarriage.[115] Toxic lead exposure is also associated with birth defects and delayed development.[116] Lead is damaging to male fertility too. According to a 1991 study, of all the toxic metals lead seems to pose the greatest threat to male fertility.[117] Research shows it can reduce sperm count, increase malformed sperm and make sperm sluggish.

Cadmium

Cadmium also negatively affects male and female fertility, according to research.[118] It is an inorganic poison present in tobacco smoke that accumulates in the body and blocks vital fertility-enhancing nutrients, such as zinc.

Aluminium

Aluminium can also seriously compromise nutritional status and therefore impact on your fertility.[119] The main sources of aluminium are antacids, deodorants, antiperspirants, anticaking ingredients found in dried milk, aluminium cookware, soft drink cans and foil.

Mercury

Mercury is a heavy, toxic metal that now contaminates the air, soil, and water in many parts of the world. Traces of mercury can be found in pesticides, dental fillings, and fish (especially tuna). The saying 'mad as a hatter' came about because hatters used to polish top hats with mercury, and many of them were poisoned by it. Mercury is extremely toxic, and studies show it can affect fertility.[120] This may be because the metal accumulates in the pituitary gland, which is vital for stimulating the production of sex hormones, and also because, according to experiments on mice in 1983, it appears to build up in the ovaries themselves. Other research links mercury with painful and irregular periods, reduced fertility rates and premature birth.

Mercury is implicated in miscarriage for workers who are exposed to it in their profession, such as dentists and factory workers who deal with mercury compounds. Women dentists have a higher rate of miscarriage, and female dental assistants exposed to mercury through the amalgam fillings they handle have been found to be less fertile than those who do not come into contact with the metal.[121] Recent research urges for the connection between mercury exposure and infertility in both men and women to be further investigated.[122,123]

If the fillings in your teeth are dark grey or silver, they contain mercury and other metals mixed together into what is called a dental amalgam. Unfortunately, mercury is poisonous, and vapours leach out of our fillings and into the body all the time, especially when we drink something hot like tea or coffee, when we brush our teeth and when we chew gum. A study of several hundred research papers and clinical reviews suggests that mercury stored in our body may cause a wide variety of symptoms, including allergies, fatigue, mood disorders, flu-like symptoms, menstrual problems, reduced sperm count, ovulation disorder's and miscarriage.[122–127]

The use of dental amalgams has been banned in both Sweden and Austria on health grounds. In Japan and Germany, though not prohibited by law, there is a high level of awareness and amalgam fillings are rarely used. In the UK the British Dental Association has not officially accepted that they are a health hazard but a growing number of private dentists are willing to help patients get rid of them.

Checklist For Avoiding Reproductive Toxins

All the chemicals and other toxic substances that we absorb in our daily life can collect in our system, make symptoms of PCOS worse and damage our fertility. There is a clear link between reproductive toxins and infertility, so it makes sense to avoid possible sources of contamination.

First of all, see if your work or home exposes you to toxic metals and then look for other possibilities:

Cleanse Your Diet

Eat nutritious food and supplement wisely. A cleansing diet, as outlined above, avoiding alcohol, and cadmium from smoking and exposure to passive smoking – all of which can have a toxic effect on the body – is the best way to avoid toxin damage.[128] You may also want to take specific nutrients (see the Diet and Detox box on page 74) to help eliminate the toxins from your system.

Lose Weight

Michel Odent, the famous French waterbirth gynaecologist, believes losing excess body fat will help as that's where we store toxins. If you are trying to lose weight this can be another great motivator.

Avoid Aluminium

Avoid aluminium kitchenware, foil and foods and indigestion tablets containing aluminium additives.

Avoid Lead

Check if your water supply has lead pipes, as lead can leach into the water just by standing in lead pipes overnight. If you have lead pipes, allow your tap to run for a minute first thing in the morning. Use water from the cold, not the hot tap because lead dissolves more easily into hot water. Also use a water filter for all your water, including cooking, hot drinks, and so on.

Avoid, where possible, heavily lead-polluted air; for example, don't stand around in heavy traffic areas. Close car windows when going through tunnels.

Check Toiletries and Cosmetics

Check labels of toiletries and cosmetics. Be especially wary of the aluminium in deodorants and antiperspirants. Use natural cosmetic products and deodorants.

Refuse Mercury Fillings

Refuse, and when possible, replace mercury-containing dental fillings. Have mercury fillings replaced with nontoxic ones. There are high levels of mercury in tuna fish, so keep your intake down to three times a week.

Check Chemicals at Work

Check what chemicals and toxins you may be exposed to at work. Carbon disulphide, used in several manufacturing processes, such as the production of plastics, has been linked to sexual dysfunction in both women and men. Many pesticides and herbicides are known reproductive toxins. People working in gardens, parks, plant nurseries and farms are at risk. Exposure to anaesthetics for health workers such as nurses and vets, to heavy metals (traffic fumes and cheap paint), to solvents (dry cleaning and lab staff), and to glycol ethers used by electronics manufacturing firms, has been linked to fertility problems in both men and women.

Computer Protection Tips

When long hours working in front of computers first started to affect women's lives, one study showed that women who spend more than 20 hours a week in front of a VDU screen such as a TV or computer monitor have twice the risk of miscarriage as those who don't.[129] This led to a lot of concern, as so many of us spend time in front of the TV or computer. But the vast majority of scientific evidence from places as diverse as the UK, Singapore, and Canada reveals there is no difference in fertility or successful pregnancy rates, regardless of how much you use a VDU.[130–131]

If you are still concerned, try these 2 useful tips:

- Switch the VDU off, rather than using the screensaver, when you are not using it.
- According to the Institute de Recherches en Geobiologie at Chardonne in Switzerland, which has investigated the effects of radiation of a variety of plants, a cactus called *Cereus peruvianus* will help absorb some of the VDU's electromagnetic radiation.

Check For House and Garden Toxins

Check what toxins you may be exposed to in your own home. Try not to use pesticides in your garden and have your house treated for woodworm when you aren't living there. Treat your pets or your house for bugs with natural herbal sprays or garlic. Be careful if you are decorating your home and avoid solvent-based paints and white spirits. Buy solvent-free paints instead and minimize the amount of chemicals you use in your home such as polish, bleach, detergents, and air fresheners. Try to buy natural products or use tried and tested cleaners like vinegar, baking soda or borax.

Check for Electromagnetic Radiation
Devices that emit electromagnetic radiation, such as VDUs, television, mobile phones, radios and microwave ovens, should also be used with caution and as far away from your bedroom as possible.

Diet and Detox

According to research by Foresight 'The preferred method of detoxification must undoubtedly be nutritional since it does not have the same potential for adverse side effects as drugs, which can remove essential elements as well as toxins.'[132]

Research backs this up. A judicious choice of food can counteract toxic substances.[133] For example, when humans consume fish that have absorbed mercury from contaminated water, selenium can act as a natural antagonist for mercury poisoning.[134] Some vegetables can accumulate cadmium from contaminated soil, and zinc found in a variety of nuts and vitamin C found in oranges and bell peppers can inhibit that conversion.[135] In addition, calcium neutralizes both lead and aluminum toxicity.[136]

Antioxidants are protective substances that patrol the body, mopping up toxins.[137] Research has shown how powerful they can be in the removal of toxins from the body. The antioxidants vitamin A, E, and C and selenium all have powerful detoxing effects.[138] Vitamin A helps to activate the enzymes needed for detoxification.[139] In one study, vitamin C along with zinc, reduced blood lead levels in psychiatric outpatients.[140] Vitamin C has also been shown to lower cadmium levels in birds. Vitamin E is such a good detoxifying agent that those with the highest intake of vitamin E (and vitamin C) have the lowest rates of cancer and heart disease. Vitamin E may also reduce lead poisoning.

As an antioxidant, selenium protects against a wide variety of degenerative diseases including liver disease.[141] Another beneficial supplement is sodium alginate.[142] This naturally occurring sea product is effective in helping to remove toxic metals. Sulfur can be important too.[143,144] Garlic, cruciferous vegetables and eggs are good sources of nutritional sulfur. In studies done with mice, cruciferous vegetables (brussel sprouts, cabbage, cauliflower and broccoli) have inhibited the induction of toxic overload and cancer. Researchers speculate that the phytochemicals in cruciferous vegetables, called isothiocyanates, help the body produce enzymes that destroy toxins.[145]

STEP SIX: ASK YOURSELF IF YOU'RE READY

Emotional health is as important for fertility as physical health. We've seen how your body is unlikely to ovulate if you aren't eating properly and, as we saw in the earlier section on stress, in a similar way your sex hormones can fail to function properly if you are unhappy or distressed.

Stresses that have been found to suppress ovulation and menstrual cycle functioning include low self-esteem, poor body image and negative or ambivalent feelings about a relationship or the prospect of motherhood. Research has even shown that in some cases women who don't ovulate can often be more tense, anxious, and have lower self-esteem compared to ovulatory women.[146,147]

With the latest scientific research showing how emotional and psychological factors can be barriers to conception, finding ways to reconnect with your inner self and really focusing on what having a child means to you can be a healing process. Niravi Payne, internationally recognized leader in mind-body fertility and founder of the Whole Person Fertility Program in Brooklyn, New York, uses exercises, meditations, visualizations and journal writing to help her clients topple any emotional barriers that may be behind their difficulty in conceiving. Niravi recognizes that there are certain conditions, such as PCOS, that can prevent a pregnancy but says, 'I have found that the vast majority of reproductive difficulties are responsive to mind-body fertility therapy.'

Without a doubt, the state of your mind and your body are connected (why else do you always go down with a cold when you feel stressed?) This isn't in any way to blame you for having PCOS. We want to emphasize that you, your partner and your body aren't in any way to blame if you have problems getting pregnant. But by becoming more aware of the connection between how you feel and what happens in your body, you may be able to influence your ability to conceive by making changes in your life.

'When my twin brother died in a car crash I was fifteen and it felt as if my arms and my legs had been cut off. I somehow stumbled through school and college and into the workplace, but a part of me was deeply wounded. I had a few disastrous relationships but then I met a guy who made me feel happy for the first time in years. We got married and started trying for a baby. When nothing happened, my doctor explained that I had PCOS and I would need fertility drugs. I had three cycles of Clomid but nothing happened. Then my husband's parents died within a few months of each other and we both felt that we needed to take a break from the treatment. My husband was very open with his grief and I watched him feel the hurt and gradually take steps to move forward with his life – something I had never done. For the first time I sat down in a heap and cried about all the hurt, the pain and the loss I felt all those years ago, when I was fifteen and didn't have the emotional resources to cope with the enormity of it all. It sounds strange but it felt good to let go, as if I had been waiting for this moment, and now I could breathe

again. A few months later I got pregnant without the help of Clomid or any other drug. You can say it was luck but I really feel that until I had let my pain and sadness for my brother go, my body wasn't ready to let a new life begin.' **JANE, 32**

What do you feel about the prospect of motherhood? Do you think you will make a good mother? Have negative feelings about yourself contributed to fertility problems? Are you ready to raise a child? It does seem that your body has a built-in mechanism to stop you getting pregnant at times when you don't feel secure or ready for a baby. If there are areas of your life where you are struggling, these can be so much harder to cope with when a baby arrives.

How Positive Are You?

It isn't always easy to know if you are under emotional strain but when they someone to describe a positive state of mind psychologists include the following:

- *Feeling okay and reasonably content*
  When you wake up in the morning how do you feel? How many times do you laugh during the day? Do you ever feel happy for no reason? Can you think of the future without feeling anxious?

- *Having stable moods and not being on a constant rollercoaster*
  How would you describe your general mood during the day? Are they fairly even or will the least little thing get you really angry?

- *Being able to connect with others but also being happy in your own company*
  Do you have people in your life, a partner, a friend, a relative, who you

can open up to or do you dread meeting people or being alone? Do you enjoy your own company or do you hate being alone?

- *Being able to give and receive love and affection.*
  Is it easy and natural for you to express physical affection?

- *Feeling your emotions fully and being able to manage them*
  Is it easy for you to allow yourself to feel strong emotions? Can you face difficult emotions like anger or do you fear them?

- *Enjoying your relationships at home and work*
  Would you say that your relationships in general are positive or are they strained? Do you enjoy your job? What's your home life like?

- *Enjoying life's simple pleasures: food, sex, exercise*
  Do you like your own body? Do you enjoy sex? Do you enjoy food and drink? Are you interested in many aspects of life and the world around you?

Everybody is different and there is no right or wrong response to the questions above, but if you suspect that right now you aren't feeling as good about yourself or your life as you could do, you may want to take stock. What do you need from the different areas of your life? Perhaps you could talk it over with someone you can trust, or a counsellor.

Is the Clock Ticking?

'For seven years now we have been trying for a baby. I'm in my early thirties, so I have got time, but I can't help thinking something is wrong with me. My partner and I are desperate for a baby. I thought getting pregnant would be so easy. Well it was for all my friends, but it wasn't *for me. The thought that I might be infertile crosses my mind, but I keep pushing it away. It makes me feel so depressed. I've recently been diagnosed with PCOS. I'm not sure whether this makes me feel better or worse. I just want to know if I will ever get to be a mother.'* SALLY, 32

You can't slow down or stop the biological clock, but this doesn't mean you have to be pressured by it. While it is true that you are working under a deadline and 35 does seem a crucial turning point for women with PCOS, it is vital that you don't panic. Panic won't help you make the best decision and, if you decide that you do want to conceive, it won't help you get pregnant either. If fears about your fertility and anxiety about whether or not you want or can have a baby are taking over your life, it is important that you visit your doctor or seek advice and support. *(See also the section on biological clock anxiety on page 214)*

STEP SEVEN: ENJOY YOUR SEX LIFE

'Sex really did lose magic and appeal when we started trying for a baby. At first we laughed about me calling John at work and saying, 'Come home now I'm ready and waiting!' but as the months passed and nothing seemed to work it actually got harder and harder to feel sexy. I just started thinking of sex as a mechanical process – rather than a way of giving and receiving pleasure. I think John felt the same – it got harder and harder for him to have erections. That, of course, made me feel that he didn't find me attractive. I didn't think that it might have something to do with the fact that in concentrating on a baby we had neglected our relationship. Later he told me that he felt like a sperm donor, not a husband.' JANET, 36

If all that you can think about is making a baby, sex can lose its spontaneity. No specific research has been done but it does seem logical from conclusions drawn by other research that enjoying lovemaking and especially having an orgasm helps to retain more active sperm.[148] The message is clear. If you want to increase your chances of conceiving, relax and enjoy sex more.

Don't Get Hung Up on Timetable Sex

One great discovery that should help to ease the pressure is that, although making love in the week before and at the time of ovulation may well help increase your chances of conception, the latest research has suggested it may not be quite as important as previously thought.[f]

A study conducted by the US National Institute of Environmental Health Sciences (NIEHS) in North Carolina suggested that fertility-day timing is far less predictable than experts had thought, which will come as a great relief to women with irregular cycles who have no idea when they ovulate. Gynaecologists have always known that ovulation day can vary a little even for women with super-regular cycles, but they never realized how often this happened and to what extent. Now the NIEHS figures suggest the possibility that, even in healthy women with no fertility problems, ovulation isn't an exact science and may only occur around day 14 in one in three women.

This has caused quite a stir among fertility experts, but where does it leave a woman with PCOS? Learning to read your ovulation signals might help (see page 35), and groundbreaking research by Canadian scientists, published in the medical journal *Fertility and Sterility* suggests that women experience far more hormonal surges each month than previously believed, all designed to create the possibility of ovulation.[149] While this might make it harder to pinpoint ovulation exactly by measuring hormones, it could lead to new ways of administering fertility treatments.

The best advice is probably the oldest advice: to maximize your chances of pregnancy have as much sex as possible. Lots of sex will help normalize your cycles and help your partner too, as the idea that abstaining from sex for up to a week so they save up sperm isn't helpful. Abstaining will stack up larger volumes of sperm but at the same time it will reduce the quality of the sperm, and poorer-quality sperm are less likely to make you pregnant, no matter how many of them there are.

'Home testing for ovulation whether by kits or temperature can be expensive and frustrating,' says Adam Balen, Professor of Reproductive Medicine and Surgery at Leeds Teaching Hospitals, the foremost reproductive gynaecologist in the UK with an interest in PCOS. 'It may be very difficult to predict ovulation and the most accurate way is through a fertility clinic performing a combination of scans and hormone tests. Regular intercourse is also important as many couples mistakenly believe that they should only have intercourse at the time of ovulation – whereas this is obviously when fertilisation occurs it isn't good for sperm to be stored in the testicles for too long and so a man should be ejaculating every 2–3 days to keep the sperm healthy.'

Don't just have sex at night-time. Fertility experts believe that the most likely time for a woman to ovulate is at 4 p.m. If you can find somewhere private to meet, an excellent time to make love would be lunchtime – it would certainly cheer up your day.

So you don't need to get obsessed with the idea of timetable sex. In fact, your body may well help you to feel more sexy at the right times, anyway – with some researchers believing that, like many animals, a desire for mating in humans is when a female ovulates. Many women say that not only do they feel more sexy but their partners feel more sexually stimulated when their wives or girlfriends are ovulating. So let nature take its course and have sex when you want to have sex – you're more likely to enjoy it then, too – and this can also bring about fertility benefits.

The Importance of Orgasm

Although a man usually needs to have an orgasm for conception to happen, it is not necessary for a woman to have one, but it can help if a woman can climax after the man because the contractions of her womb and vagina create a partial vacuum, which will help to suck the sperm up into her cervix. Without orgasm they will still get there, just not so quickly.

Research suggests that orgasm is a sophisticated way for women to select unconsciously which lover's sperm is used to increase the chances of conception.[150] Two British biologists, Robin Baker and Mark Bellis, discovered that when a woman climaxes anytime between 1 minute before to 45 minutes after her lover ejaculates, she retains significantly more sperm than she does after nonorgasmic sex. In addition, their research results indicated that the strong muscular contractions associated with orgasm pull sperm from the vagina to the cervix, where it's in a better position to reach an egg. So it appears that on a physiological level orgasm in women serves to favour the man she feels would make the best father to her child.

Satisfying Sex

Research also shows that women who have regular satisfying sex, with intercourse at least once a week, have more regular menstrual cycles and fewer fertility problems than those who don't.[151] In addition, a satisfying sex life can be a wonderful way to reduce stress and therefore encourage fertility. How? In much the same way as exercise reduces body tension that can interfere with hormone production, so can sex. The tension-releasing power of orgasm can be so great for some people that its effects are more powerful than a tranquillizer.

A loving, caring, emotionally supportive relationship can also have a positive effect on your fertility. Women can spontaneously ovulate when they fall in love and there is growing evidence that, when you feel happy and secure and loved and have a fulfilling sex life, fertility can prosper. This isn't to say that being single, or having an argument or break up will affect your fertility, or that a bad relationship can't produce a baby, but if your love life is chronically stressful it may contribute to your fertility problems.

Does it Matter Who's on Top?

With all this good news about how regular, enjoyable sex is the best way to boost fertility, why not turn that into an opportunity to experiment with a few positions to up the fertility levels even more?

Are there ways you can make love to help you conceive? Yes, says fertility expert Dr Niels Lauersen, an obstetrician/gynaecologist with the St Vincent Medical Center in New York City. He believes that, 'the positions both you and your partner assume during and right after making love can significantly affect the passage of sperm into your vagina to your fallopian tube.'

Many experts believe that the man-on-top position has the best chance of getting a woman pregnant, but there are no studies to prove this. The rationale is that this position allows for deep penetration so the man's sperm can be ejaculated as close to the cervix as possible. This gives the sperm cells a flying start on their long journey, as the closer they are to the ripe egg waiting in the fallopian tube several centimeters further up in a woman's body, the more likely they are to reach it. Logically, any position that goes against gravity, such as woman on top or having sex sitting or standing up, discourages the sperm's journey upward and is thought to deter conception.

If a man enters a woman from behind, especially if she is kneeling in front of him so she is at an angle with her bottom higher than her head, it is said to encourage conception. Making love in the spoons position (both partners facing the same way with the man penetrating the woman from behind) is not thought to be such an effective baby-making position because the penetration angle is not so deep. The chances might be maximized if the woman leans the upper half of her body a little away from her partner, pushing her bottom against him.

Studies show that the best and fittest sperm have reached the fallopian tube in five minutes and the rest usually get there within 45 minutes.[152] So as long as you don't leap up or go to the toilet the moment you are finished, you probably don't need to be stuck on the floor or bed with one eye on the clock. In any case, it is the fastest and fittest sperm that you want to fertilize the egg. In the words of Dr Steve Brody of the Advanced Fertility Institute in San Diego, 'The sperm that get in there right away have the best chance of fertilizing the egg. A study in rabbits shows that if you destroy all sperm in the vagina within five minutes, the rabbit can still get pregnant.'

No Sex Please – I'm Tired

It's all very well knowing you should be having regular sex in all sorts of fun positions – but what if you're too stressed and too tired? Dr Rosalind Bramwell, fertility researcher from the University of Liverpool says that 'not being interested anymore is something that many couples don't like to admit to. Even to themselves.'

A new condition called TINS is a real threat to fertility rates. It stands for Two Incomes No Sex. According to research by a British organization called the Chartered Institute of Personnel and Development, over half the people they interviewed said their sex lives were suffering because of the long hours they spent at work, which meant they felt too tired at the end of the day.

Good sex lasts minutes not hours!

Sometimes it can be easy to feel that to make time for sex in a busy life, you need to put aside a whole evening. But satisfactory sexual intercourse for couples lasts from 3 to 13 minutes, contrary to popular fantasy about the need for hours of sexual activity, according to a survey of US and Canadian sex therapists.[153]

I'm Not In The Mood

> 'I really want to start a family with my partner but we haven't had sex for about a year now. I really feel sorry for him and he has a lot to put up with, but when I'm gaining weight, losing hair and feeling spotty and grotty because of PCOS, the last thing on my mind is sex. I'm just never in the mood.' ANNA, 30

If you never seem to feel in the mood for sex and your libido is low you aren't in the minority. In the February 1999 issue of the *Journal of the American Medical Association*, Researchers reported on the sexual health of Americans and revealed that 43 percent of American women suffer from sexual dysfunction and loss of libido. They noted that the 'experience of sexual dysfunction is more likely among women with poor physical and emotional health and overall wellbeing.' Poor health and lifestyle impair sexual drive and desire.

You may wonder why this is important. The answer is threefold. First, whether you have PCOS or not, if you're in a relationship, lack of sexual desire is upsetting and likely to leave your mate in a state of confusion, embarrassment or feeling inadequate. Second, whether you have PCOS or not, if you don't have a fulfilling sex life, you're missing out on one of life's great pleasures. And third – again whether you have PCOS or not – sex is good for your health.

Think your way to desire

If you've had a bad day, you're tired, or overwhelmed with the demands of kids, work, and life, this visualisation exercise from psychotherapist Jules McClean (www.julesmccleancounselling. co.uk), is designed to energise you, and encourage your adrenaline and sexual appetite to kick in.

Find 5 to 10 minutes (on your journey home, when you get home from work, when your partner is out and about), then sit comfortably, and breathe deeply in and out 10–20 times. On the out breath visualise stress fluttering away from your body.

Next, think about the parts of your body you like and how it might feel to be touched there. Allow yourself to give in to the fantasy of being held, stroked, kissed and caressed by your partner and think about where you might like to touch him. Imagine your ideal place for a sexual encounter – whether it's in your house, a hotel, an isolated beach or a steamy tropical forest. Feel the textures (crisp linen, soft sand), taste the tension, smell the aromas, and let your mind help your body feel sensual.

Yes, it's true PCOS can make it harder for you to feel sexy but it's important to understand that PCOS alone probably isn't the reason for loss of libido. For one, the hormone imbalance in PCOS isn't necessarily to blame, as raised testosterone should, in theory, increase your sex drive (testosterone therapy is becoming much more common as a libido-booster for menopausal women). So what's going on? As well as the possibility of poor physical and emotional health, if you aren't getting enough nutrients in your diet or exercising enough, or are feeling low, libido is one of the first things to suffer. But as we've seen in the fertility-boosting plan there are steps you can take to improve your physical and emotional health. And by taking these steps towards a healthier you the chances are your libido will improve too.

It can take a month or two to really feel the benefits of the fertility boosting plan, so here are some reminders and ideas in the meantime:

Give Your Sex Life a Kick-Start

- Do eat healthily according to the guidelines in our plan. Vitamin A and B zinc and selenium are all crucial for libido; and exercise helps too, by boosting your mood and body image.

- Check your stress levels. 'In general, stress dampens libido. A stressed woman may blame a host of other factors for her symptoms, without realizing that stress is the real cause of the problem,' says Milwaukee urologist and sex therapist Dr Stuart Fine. Deal with commonplace stress by following the de-stressing tips on page 40.

- Go with it. Even if you feel tired, sluggish, stressed or just 'not in the mood', you can still create and enjoy a fulfilling sexual experience. 'One of the many myths of "movie sex" is that both people are turned-on before touching even begins,' says Professor of Psychology Barry W. McCarthy, author of *Enduring Desire*. In fact, most people have to allow themselves to get in the mood as the sexual connection begins. In the same way as we can make ourselves cry by watching a sad movie, or make ourselves turned on by reading an erotic book, we can find desire by slowly melting into an experience. 'The most important thing,' says sexual and relationship psychotherapist Paula Hall, author of

Improving your Sexual Relationship for Dummies, 'is not to want to, but to want to want to.'

- Depression is another major inhibitor of sexual desire. Try to understand why you are feeling low, so that you act appropriately when low feelings come. If you feel you can't cope alone, reach out for the support of family and friends or see your doctor for referral to a counsellor or therapist.

- Most sex therapists agree that sex begins in the head – in a way it's an idea that overtakes you. Your body's physical reaction follows. A key part of starting that sexual idea is setting the mood and romantic music can help, as can low lighting, a candlelit bath, or your favourite romantic or raunchy film. If you haven't felt sexy for a while, touching yourself can also be a way to reconnect with your body as a sensual, sexual pleasure. Once you're back in touch with your own desires, it can be easier and less daunting to connect with your partner's.

- Re-evaluate how you feel about your body. Remind yourself that your ability to become aroused, achieve sexual satisfaction and reciprocate is there no matter what you weigh or look like. Stop focusing on what society tells you is beautiful and concentrate instead on what you find beautiful and pleasurable about yourself.

- Relationship troubles can also contribute to loss of sexual desire. If you don't feel listened to, respected or important, it is natural to respond with resentment and that resentment can dampen libido. It's important to open the lines of communication with your partner so that anger can be expressed in places other than the bedroom. If the problem is severe, such as infidelity, you may want to go to a relationship counsellor.

- If you find the idea of sex unappealing or uncomfortable, talk to a sex therapist to discuss your health, your upbringing, yourcircumstances, any body image issues you may have and your relationship, so that you can find ways to give yourself permission to satisfy your sexual needs. You may want to do this alone or you may find that it is more productive to talk to a sex therapist with your partner.

- Make time for romance. Give it a higher priority in your life. However busy or stressful your life gets, try to make sure that you have some 'couple time' where you can unwind together and talk about your day. Plan regular meals out, cinema trips or weekend breaks so that the two of you get some special time together away from the hustle and bustle of your daily life.

- Nature provides many safe, natural ways to boost sexual desire. Certain foods, such as chocolate, figs and ginger are thought to contain aphrodisiac qualities because they contain nutrients that are essential for boosting libido. Any food that contains zinc, such as nuts or oysters, could be considered an aphrodisiac, as zinc is thought to have a positive effect on libido.

- Aromatherapists suggest that certain scents can have an aphrodisiac effect. Michelle Roques-O'Neil (see Resource Guide on page 275 for details) produces a passion blend, containing jasmine, rose, patchouli and sandalwood. This blend, which is uplifting and sensual, can be used in the bath, as a massage oil or dabbed on your pulse points. Smell works through association too.[154] Returning to a perfume you used to wear when you first met your partner may rekindle the passion.

- Massage can also help relax and invigorate. Treat yourself to a massage or treat your partner to one. California-based Robert Tisserand, founder of Tisserand Aromatherapy, suggests a sensual massage with the following oils: 30 drops of sweet almond oil, five drops of ylang-ylang, four drops of lavender and three drops of jasmine.

Keep Your Cool

You've probably heard stories of couples who tried really hard to get pregnant and only conceived when they gave up. Hence the notion of trying too hard continues to be perpetuated – yes, but only when trying turns from a natural loving desire to have a baby into a demand filled with anxiety, fear and worry, which are the real culprits.

Feel calm and confident about your sexuality and your ability to become a mother. Whether you have PCOS or not, maintaining the right emotional state is perhaps one of the best ways to enjoy your sex life and achieve conception. Make healthy diet and lifestyle choices as our plan suggests but above all relax, stay calm, make love…enjoy.

THAT'S THE LAST STEP…WHAT NEXT?

The seven-step plan is a lot to take in all in one go – so don't expect to be able to make the changes overnight. Ideally, you should be putting it in place over three or four months to give yourself and your partner a chance to get into the habit of following these guidelines, so they just become second nature. This isn't a 'miracle' cure that will have you pregnant overnight – but you'll be amazed at how many women with PCOS have reported positive improvements in their symptoms, and have got pregnant after getting their diets, emotions and lifestyles into shape. So take a deep breath and be patient – stick to the plan and you might be surprised at how dramatic the results are.

However, if you've been following the plan and you still have some problems to iron out – from irregular periods to unexplained non-conception – then it's time to move on to our fine-tuning chapter to tackle those issues.

Chapter Three

. . . .

Tackling Stubborn PCOS Problems:
Fine-tuning Your Self-Help Programme

So you've been following the seven-step plan in the previous section of this book, and you're still having some problems. Whether you just want to get your body into its best shape for a possible pregnancy some time in the future, or whether you've been trying for a while and the long-awaited pregnancy hasn't yet happened, it's time to look for some more solutions. Don't give up the seven steps, though – they are your basic foundation plan for boosting your fertility, and the advice in this section is designed to be used on top of that to give you the added oomph you need to conceive.

The general advice given to couples considering a pregnancy is to try for a year or two and if nothing happens to come back but, if you have PCOS, waiting any more than six months is bad advice, and if it comes from your doctor find another one. 'If you have PCOS, think you have PCOS, or have irregular periods, don't wait a year to have the diagnosis of infertility. Seek help earlier,' urges PCOS expert Dr Samuel Thatcher. This is especially true if you're 35 or over as fertility naturally starts to decline at this age.

So now's the time to see your doctor for a health screen. Getting a thorough check up for you and your partner, to check sperm counts or investigate for blocked fallopian tubes or infections, is a really good thing to do. You may as well get all this checked out now so you know you are going forward with every possible chance of maximizing your fertility.

GETTING YOUR PARTNER'S FERTILITY CHECKED

When presenting for fertility treatment, your doctor or fertility specialist will ask for your partner's sperm to be checked too. If the sperm is abnormal he may be referred to a urologist or an andrologist, but a reproductive endocrinologist will be the best person to explain options and coordinate efforts. A question you should always ask when selecting a clinic is whether or not the team includes a reproductive urologist or an andrologist.

Don't be surprised if your partner gets anxious when asked for a semen sample at a fertility clinic. For a man to be told he has abnormal or poorly performing sperm is equivalent to a women being told she can not carry a child. Men equate sperm counts with virility and manliness and infertility can attack the male self-image as strongly as that of the female.

What Can He Do to Improve His Fertility?

'Women with PCOS often share lifestyle evils with their partners,' says Dr Thatcher, 'and there is no better way than to work on the problems together.' As we saw in the previous chapter, there is a close link between male obesity and decreased testosterone. Smoking, caffeine and poor diet can affect sperm count, as can alcohol and certain medications. There is also the theory that increased heat can reduce sperm count. Without a doubt, research suggests that diet and lifestyle changes can have a positive effect on sperm count.

WHAT NEXT?

If you and your partner have been given a clean bill of health, and if you and your doctor have identified that PCOS is definitely the problem, you can use the following self-help strategies to help you overcome your particular issues, from irregular periods to overweight; or you can use these self-help strategies alongside fertility treatment if this is the course of action you and your healthcare provider decide is right. Taking these extra steps on top of your basic fertility-boosting lifestyle plan will increase your chances of success on an orthodox fertility programme. Select the problem you want to focus on and use the advice to crank up your fertility another notch.

STUBBORN PROBLEM ONE: IRREGULAR PERIODS

'I don't think I've ever had a regular menstrual cycle. It didn't worry me before but, now that I'm thinking of starting a family, it does. I have a period only two or three times a year and I'm worried about my fertility.'
REBECCA, **30**

'I'm 26 and I've never had a period. It was horrible at school when all my friends started. When I got to 14 and nothing happened I just pretended I had, and even went so far as to wear sanitary towels in PE lessons so they wouldn't suspect I was lying.' MARY, **26**

For most women with PCOS concerned about their fertility, irregular periods are probably the most common problem and for good reason.[155] The main issue is the regularity of a woman's cycle,' says Adam Balen, 'the less regular, the greater reduction in fertility.'

Regular cycles are usually 23 to 35 days apart, but as long as your periods occur at roughly the same time each cycle – for example, they could be 45 days apart, instead of the typical 28, but they always appear around day 45 – they are classified as being regular. 'In reality,' says Toni

Weschler, fertility awareness counsellor and author of *Taking Charge of Your Fertility*, 'cycles vary tremendously among women and often within each woman herself.' This is because our bodies are affected by so many things, from diet, to stress or medication.

If your periods are regular and your cycle length is less than 35 days from one bleed to the next, there is a greater than 95 percent chance that you are ovulating, according to Dr Adam Balen. (This, of course, isn't the case if you are on the pill. The pill suppresses ovulation and the bleeds you have when on the pill do not signify regular ovulation.) If there are long gaps between your periods and then you have a heavy period, this could mean that you aren't ovulating, as lack of ovulation is a common cause of heavy bleeding.

What Qualifies as Irregular Periods?

If you have irregular periods you simply don't know when your period is going to come,' says Dr Helen Mason 'You have no idea when and if you are ovulating – even a slightly irregular cycle means that timing intercourse is harder.' The following symptoms are typical:

- Large gaps with no periods

- Some gaps, then periods coming too quickly, or bleeding continuously for a few weeks

- Spotting in between periods.

It can be disconcerting not to have regular periods – as Linda, 34, says, 'It's a weird feeling, kind of like when you need to sneeze but can't. I can't explain but it just doesn't feel right.' There is no need to worry about backed-up periods, or the idea that there's a build-up of blood in your body because it isn't being shed every month.

'Rest assured,' says Dr Geoffrey Redmond, Department of Pediatric Endocrinology, New York Hospital, Cornell Medical Center, 'that lack of menstruation does not result in an accumulation of toxins in your body.' Amenorrhoea, the medical term given to absent periods, does not involve the backing up of menstrual fluid, because the menstrual fluid isn't being formed at all.

So how does this interfere with fertility – after all, you don't have periods when you're pregnant! The problem is that your womb usually only sheds its lining if ovulation has taken place during the cycle. Your period is actually triggered by an egg being released, as its empty follicle then pumps out progesterone in the second half of your cycle, and this eventually reaches a level that causes your womb lining to shed as a period. So if you're not cycling, chances are you're not ovulating – and that's the reason you're not getting pregnant.

What Can You Do About It?

First, you need to look beyond your PCOS for a moment. Although irregular periods are a common symptom of PCOS, they're also caused by lots of other day-to-day things – and you need to rule those out before you focus all your energy on fine-tuning your PCOS self-care programme.

Crash dieting, stress, seasonal changes, travel (especially long distance air travel), heavy exercise and illness can all cause a disruption in your cycle and usually periods return when full health is recovered and stress is reduced.[156] For example, as we explained in the previous chapter, if you don't have enough fat stores because of dieting, exercise or weight loss, your body will think that you're starving. Since it's not appropriate to get pregnant when food is scarce, research has shown that your body will simply shut down your menstrual cycle. Periods will stop or become irregular until you get your fat stores back.[157]

In a similar way, when under stress your body reacts to the crisis by affecting your menstrual cycle – nature's way of protecting you from pregnancy when it's less likely you will cope. It's well known that women going through a bereavement or any other kind of major trauma can stop menstruating. 'You can't fool your body,' says Sarah Berga MD, Associate Professor of Obstetrics, Gynecology and Psychiatry at the University of Pittsburgh. 'Your body knows. It makes a judgement call. It knows that it is under stress and since it won't have enough energy to maintain vital functioning it gets rid of the reproductive cycle until health has been restored.'

The odd skipped period or late period isn't anything to panic about, but it is a warning sign. Your body is trying to tell you that you are not 100 percent well. But if you have had irregularities for more than three cycles, or if your periods have simply stopped altogether, the likely cause isn't stress or an upset in your routine but PCOS, according to Dr James Douglas, reproductive endocrinologist from the Plano Medical Center in Texas. (Do bear in mind, though, that other conditions, such as fibroids, thyroid disorders, infection, eating disorders and chronic illness, can all cause menstrual irregularity. If you have any of these, or suspect they could be playing a part, ask your doctor to rule them out.)

Why Does PCOS Cause Irregular Periods?

As we explained in the first chapter, the menstrual cycle in women with PCOS is often irregular because you can't have a period without ovulation – and in some women with PCOS, the eggs are not being developed and released owing to the wrong balance of hormones in the body.

It seems that in women with PCOS, follicles start to mature but for some reason fail to ripen properly or to be released. Instead, they stay in the ovaries and continue to produce oestrogen but no progesterone. Remember, progesterone is the hormone that prepares your body for pregnancy if an egg is fertilized by a sperm, or for menstruation if no egg is fertilized. Over time, more and more trapped follicles build up so that the ovaries become filled with the empty egg follicles, which are known as cysts, and hard fibrotic growths, which show up on an ultrasound screen.

This pattern could continue for many months and for some women with PCOS it does. They can go for 2 to 24 months or more without a period. For other women the lining of the womb, which has become overgrown due to oestrogen production, begins to break down of its own accord and they experience spotting or heavy bleeding. In some cases a follicle does eventually manage to develop and ovulation occurs and a new cycle begins.

'Unfortunately, there are still no clear answers as to why this happens,' says Dr Douglas. 'All we do know is that there are problems in the hormonal feedback loop that regulates the menstrual cycle.' Elevated levels of luteinizing hormone (LH) and ooestrogen have been found in some but not all women with PCOS and this can block ovulation.[158] Research by Professor Franks, Professor of Reproductive Enocrinology at Imperial College, London, has shown that higher than normal levels of the hormone testosterone are also associated with PCOS and irregular periods.[159] Testosterone inhibits ovulation. Research has also focused on why some women with PCOS have higher than normal levels of insulin.[160,161] It is possible that elevated levels of insulin encourage testosterone production by the ovaries and contribute to menstrual disturbances. But the general consensus is that inappropriate levels of LH, oestrogen, insulin and testosterone are, again, symptoms rather than causes of PCOS – the root cause or causes remain as yet unknown.

So, How Can I Tell If I'm Ovulating?

It is possible to have periods and not to ovulate but generally regular periods are a good indication that you are ovulating – even if you only have four or five periods a year. If your periods are irregular the chances are you aren't ovulating (see also page 35 in Chapter Two).

Ovulation Predictor Kits

You might be tempted to buy an ovulation predictor kit from your chemist. The kits contain a simple dipstick urine test that you can do at home. They work by detecting the surge of LH hormone, which happens 24 to 36 hours before ovulation, but women with PCOS often have higher than normal levels of LH so it wouldn't be wise to rely on the kits because you will get inaccurate results. Also, if your periods are irregular you can never be sure when ovulation occurs, so you could end up buying lots of kits and spending a lot of money.

The Fertile Mucus Sign

'Your body gives you conspicuous signs,' says Toni Weschler, 'to help you understand on a daily basis what is transpiring within.' Certain key signals occur to suggest that ovulation – and your peak fertility time – are near and it is probably better for women with PCOS to learn to read these signs. The fertile mucus sign is the most important indicator as you may find that you don't experience any of the others.

So what is fertile mucus? This is clear, watery, stretchy mucus, like the white of runny egg. This is the most important fertility signal of all, and the easiest to detect. Note: If you have a vaginal infection, like thrush, you may not be able to detect fertility signals.

Other Signs of Ovulation

- Feeling sexier: Some women say they feel more sexy around ovulation.

- Ovulation pain: There may be a dull ache or twinge on one side of the abdomen, low down, that lasts for a few moments or a whole day.

- Softer cervix: It feels less firm and softer than usual if you touch it gently with your finger.

- Spotting: A tiny loss of blood can sometimes occur at ovulation. If you notice it chat with your doctor and make sure your cervix is healthy before linking to ovulation.

- Temperature: Body temperature drops slightly before ovulation and increases by about 0.2°C (0.4°F) afterwards. Temperature checking can seem quite complicated and it usually takes a few months to get the hang of it. It may be best to see a natural family planning counsellor who can help you learn this method.

What Choices Do I Have Now?

In order for you to have a normal menstrual cycle where ovulation does occur you need to get your hormones back in balance. Your doctor will probably suggest the contraceptive pill or metformin (see Glossary) to regulate your periods but neither of these gets to the root of the problem, the real reason why your periods are irregular. For example, the pill will regularize your cycle, but pill bleeds are not real bleeds. They are withdrawal bleeds from the effects of the pill, so when you come off the pill, symptoms that have been suppressed by the pill are likely to return. And you certainly can't get pregnant if you're on it.

There is a lot of dispute on PCOS discussion boards about whether metformin, the insulin sensitiser, which was hoped to be a real boost for women with PCOS struggling with weight loss. Even at the time when the first investigations were being carried out, experts sounded a word of warning. 'Just be aware that metformin is not a magic bullet – it won't work long term to lower insulin resistance if diet and exercise plans are not in place,' said Gerard Conway, a consultant gynaecologist at Middlesex Hospital, London.

Although some women who have been prescribed the drug may disagree, the latest expert view is that Metformin does not help weight loss, which could boost fertility in obese women with PCOS.

'We and others have done lots of research now on metformin,' says Professor Adam Balen. 'It does not achieve weight loss or enhance fertility and should only be given to women with impaired glucose tolerance (IGT) or Type 2 diabetes mellitus. But in IVF it appears to decrease risk of OHSS [ovarian hyperstimulation syndrome] so may have a role.' (For more on IVF and getting the best from it, see page 150).

You can encourage hormonal balance and therefore a more regular cycle with self-care strategies.

Improve Your Diet

Improve your diet, using the guidelines outlined in the seven-step fertility-boosting plan in the previous section of this book. We can't stress enough how many women have written to us after using our PCOS diet book to say it's helped them back to health, especially by restoring lost periods. Healthy eating can seem like a chore but don't get stressed – if you manage to stick to the rules 80 percent of the time you're doing really well. If you're still finding your periods are unpredictable, try these extra five steps to kick-start them, as research shows that blood sugar and hormone-balancing dietary approaches can really help.[162,163]

One: Keep Your Blood Sugar Balanced

Eat the right carbs — complex, low Glycemic Index foods such as vegetables, wholegrain bread, basmati rice and pulses. The Glycemic Index is a guideline for diabetics that measures the impact a food has on blood sugar when eaten. Foods with high values, such as sugar, bananas, white bread and corn chips, should be avoided and preference given to low GI foods such as legumes, beans, apples and oatmeal. To find out more, chat to your doctor and ask for a list of GI foods. Cutting down on sugar and refined white flour products will also help. This ensures healthy insulin and blood sugar levels and also helps you feel fuller for longer, to prevent overeating. Always eat breakfast and have small, frequent meals throughout the day (or three main meals and two healthy snacks), no more than three hours apart to avoid rapid fluctuations in blood sugar. Eat a little protein and fibre with each meal to slow down your body's release of sugar into your bloodstream and keep insulin levels stable.

Two: Eat Phytoestrogens

Phytoestrogens have been shown to have a balancing effect on hormones and periods.[164] Phytoestrogens are found in all fruit, vegetables and cereals but they are most beneficial in the form of isoflavones, which are found in legumes such as soya, lentils and beans, chickpeas, and garlic. These foods have a mild oestrogenic effect and can help balance levels of oestrogen because their phtyoestrogen molecules bond to the body's own oestrogen receptors. The phtyoestrogens are only weak in comparison to the body's own oestrogens — so they can help where there is excess oestrogen, as in anovulatory (no ovulation) PCOS; or when an oestrogen boost is needed, for example after menopause. Phytoestrogens also have been found to stimulate the production of sex hormone-binding globulin (SHBG). SHBG is a protein produced by the liver that binds sex hormones like oestrogen in order to control how many of them are circulating in your blood. Having the right balance of SHBG gives you a better chance of hormone balance.[165]

The phytochemical DIM (indole-3-carbinol or IC3), found in cruciferous vegetables, may also have a beneficial effect on your cycle by helping to regulate oestrogen, but, because it isn't helpful if your testosterone levels are high, more research needs to be done to see if it is a suitable treatment for women with PCOS.[166]

How Much Soya?

Soy has been in and out of the news with science, with the soy industry, nutritionists, vegetarians and consumers all wanting to know whether it's good or bad for you, as conflicting advice comes to light. So what's the lowdown? In essence, eating soy in moderation, in its natural form, avoiding supplements and choosing soya beans themselves (canned or frozen are great in a Thai or Indian curry, casserole, soup or stir fry). Miso, tofu or organic soy milk is not a problem – although women may want to avoid it around the time of ovulation, and both men and women may want to reduce the amount they eat if they are overweight or obese. The reasons? Read on...

Soy and thyroid function

The good news is that the latest research on whether soy disrupts thyroid function shows it doesn't – a 3-year trial, completed in 2010, giving the soy isoflavone genistein to post-menopausal women revealed no problems.[167]

'Soy doesn't disrupt thyroid function in those with normal

thyroid function and adequate iodine,' says Dr Christiane Northrup (www.drnorthrup.com). 'The relationship between soy and thyroid function has been studied for more than 70 years. Since then, 14 human clinical trials have studied the effects of soy foods and soy isoflavones on thyroid function. All involved presumably healthy subjects, and with few exceptions, the soy product used was isolated soy protein. With only one exception, all of the studies showed either no effects or minor and clinically irrelevant effects of soy on thyroid function. The one trial that noted marked anti-thyroid effects (and the one that is often cited in anti-soy literature), involved Japanese adults who were fed roasted soybeans that had been pickled and stored in rice vinegar. It is not known what the soy protein or isoflavone content of this food was. And the study was not controlled. So no firm conclusion can be drawn.

'Most experts agree that soy foods and isolated soy protein have little if any effect on thyroid function in normal, healthy adults who consume soy at moderate levels as part of a well balanced diet. However, soy isoflavones, especially in high doses, can disrupt thyroid function in those who are iodine deficient (estimated to be 13% of the population), and in those who have compromised thyroid function.'[168]

Soy and sperm health

There have been numerous studies looking at the effects of high doses of soy on male fertility.[169–171] High doses seem to be linked with a temporary reduction in sperm count but over the course of a few days this rises again. Overweight men also seem to have a more pronounced sensitivity to the oestrogenic effects of high doses of soy isoflavones. However, when commenting on one of these studies for the BBC, Dr Allan Pacey, a senior lecturer in andrology from the

University of Sheffield, said that if soy genuinely had a detrimental effect on sperm production, fertility might well be affected in those regions of the world where it was a staple part of the diet, and there was no evidence that this was the case. This could partly reflect the fact that studies use high doses of concentrated isoflavones which do not get replicated when people eat moderate amounts of natural soy foods.

Soy and female fertility

Reducing the amount of soya you eat around ovulation could be worth a try, according to a study in humans by Professor Lynn Fraser, from King's College London, who said even tiny doses in the female tract could sabotage the sperm as it swims towards the egg, findings that she presented at the 2005 European Society for Human Reproduction and Embryology Conference.[172] And further investigation is being carried out into the effects of high soya isoflavone doses on the implantation of embryos and their subsequent development on mice.[173] Bear in mind that research in labs is done on isolated compounds given in large doses – so moderation is key, as are natural, non-processed soya products.

Other useful advice, from Dr Fiona McCulloch BSc ND (www. drfiona.whitelotusclinic.ca), a Naturopathic Physician in private practice in Toronto, a member of the Canadian Fertility and Andrology Society and specializes in Fertility, Women's Health and Hormonal Conditions, is as follows:

- Keeping your body mass index in the healthy range is key – especially as the effect of soy on overweight men has been seen to be intensified. Plus, countries such as Japan, where soya is eaten in quantity, yet birth rates are not falling, do not have a problem with obesity in the same way as the US or UK.

- Millions of women have consumed soy products and become pregnant, so it is not something to worry excessively about. Stress can have much more profound effects on your fertility than a small amount of soy.
- Genetic modification has not been considered in these studies. If you do choose to include soy in your diet, use non-GMO. Soy can also be sprayed with pesticides which often have estrogenic effects, so choose organic soy.

Four: Choose Healthy Fats

Make sure you're avoiding saturated fats from mainly animal and full-fat dairy products by choosing skimmed versions, cutting fat off your meat or using low-fat cooking methods like grilling. This is because saturated fats block your body's absorption of essential fatty acids and stimulate oestrogen production, which isn't helpful if you have irregular periods.[174]

But don't cut fat out altogether – some fats are essential for every cell in your body and are crucial to help regulate your periods by balancing your hormones. The UK Department of Health suggests that we should double our intake of omega 3 EFAs by eating oily fish two or three times a week. Other sources of omega 3 include nuts and seeds and linseed (flaxseed) oil, and also to some extent pumpkin seeds, walnuts, and dark green veggies. Research has shown that women taking 10 g of ground linseed per day increase the regularity of their cycle and improve ovulation.[175] Linseeds also have a phytoestrogenic effect – eat them sprinkled on cereal, baked in bread or added to salads or soups; or just as a teaspoon a day supplement.

Five: Use Proven Nutritional Supplements

Remember that supplements are not a substitute for a healthy diet.

Ideally you should see a nutritional therapist or dietician to make up a prescription for you. 'Eating healthily and gently detoxing your diet are the priority if you have irregular periods and PCOS. Supplements should be seen as a way to support these positive changes. A nutritionist would typically recommend a good multivitamin and mineral supplement, along with an antioxidant complex and essential fatty acid supplement for women with PCOS and irregular periods,' says nutritional expert Dr Adam Carey.

If you're not already doing so, take his advice – make sure the supplement contains vitamin B6, which has been linked to improved ovulatory rates resulting in pregnancy, and magnesium, as a deficiency in this has been linked to irregular cycles.[176,177] This multivitamin also needs to contain zinc at 30 mg per day as this is a crucial mineral for the menstrual cycle and fertility. You may also want to boost your healthy diet further with a good antioxidant formula. Also essential fatty acids – good amounts of omega 3 and omega 6 essential oils – have been proven to help regulate the cycle; nutritionist Marilyn Glenville advises supplementing with 150 g of omega 6 and at least 2 g of omega 3 per day. (See page 48 for more on these vitamins and minerals)

Keep Blood Sugar Cravings at Bay

Finding it hard to stay off the sugary snacks? You'll really help yourself to better health and fertility if you can cut down. So identify your triggers. Are there certain places, like supermarkets or parties; or certain emotions, like fear and anger; or certain activities, like watching TV, which make you reach for a chocolate bar? The more you become aware of your triggers the more you can start to deal with them. When the craving starts, try doing something else instead. For example, take a walk or do some gardening.

If you get the urge to eat, ride it out. Food cravings peak and subside like waves. When you get the craving tell yourself that you can satisfy it if you need to. Then wait a few moments. Most cravings only last a few moments. Try doing something to distract yourself.

- Don't go shopping when you are hungry – you'll end up buying sugary snacks.

- Stock up on healthy snacks – fruit with a handful of nuts, low-fat crackers with low-fat cottage cheese, vegetable sticks – and have them close at hand or in your fridge for when temptation strikes.

- Explore your health food shop. Rice cakes with bananas or pure fruit spread or peanut butter make delicious snacks.

- For a comfort fix make yourself a hot chocolate with skimmed or soya milk, or some oatmeal porridge with honey.

- Smelling vanilla essence oil can prevent cravings for sweet foods, according to research from St George's Hospital London. Drop some essence on a tissue and inhale when you feel the need.[178,179]

Take Extra Care of Your Liver

If you're following the detox guidelines in the seven-step plan you're a step ahead already in terms of detoxing, but to get on top of irregular periods it may be worth giving your liver some extra TLC. Your liver detoxifies harmful toxins and waste products. It also processes hormones that your body doesn't need anymore. For example, it deals with excess oestrogen so it can be eliminated from your body. If the liver isn't functioning well, old hormones left over from each menstrual cycle can accumulate and, if not deactivated by the liver, they can return to the bloodstream and cause trouble. Make sure that you eliminate any substances that can compromise your liver, especially alcohol. You may also want to supplement with B vitamins because they are essential for your liver to process oestrogen. The herb milk thistle is also excellent for the liver. Studies have shown how it can increase the number of new liver cells to replace old, worn out ones.[180]

STUBBORN PROBLEM TWO: NEEDING TO LOSE SOME WEIGHT

As we saw in the fertility-boosting plan, weight management is key for good health and fertility if you have PCOS – but it's often one of the most tricky aspects to get right and can feel very frustrating as PCOS tends to make weight gain easy and weight loss harder. As we stressed in the previous chapter, research has shown that weight problems are four times more likely if you have PCOS and irregular periods than if you don't, yet research has shown that weight management can trigger ovulation and regular cycles in women who have stopped ovulating.[181–183]

Following the weight management guidelines already outlined is a good start – and if you feel you need an extra boost here are some more options for you:

Ditch Faddy Diets!

'It's really unfair, but women with PCOS just don't seem to burn off calories as most people do,' says Dr Helen Mason, Senior Lecturer in Reproductive Endocrinology at St George's Hospital Medical School in London. But don't be tempted by faddy diet plans that promise fast weight loss, as they won't help you – or your fertility – in the long run.

Crash dieting is the biggest no-no if you have PCOS, as it just sends your body into starvation mode and sends your insulin metabolism into an even worse state – and sudden weight loss can actually stop your periods, too.

And what about those high protein, low or no carbohydrate diets that are widely recommended? Two studies presented to the Endocrine Society meeting in San Francisco in June 2002 suggest that so-called 'low carbing' isn't helpful for long-term health, if you have PCOS, as you end up eating high fat, low nutrient foods, which don't give you the nutrients, fibre or essential fats that you need for hormonal health and a healthy heart (you want to be around for when your kid(s) grow up, after all!). It's cutting calories by replacing sugar and high fat food with nutritious food, and increasing activity levels that matters – as we stress with our advice in the seven-step fertility boosting plan in the previous chapter. Don't throw out that sound healthy eating advice if you're finding weight loss hard – stick to protein with every meal and choose the right, low GI carbs such as vegetables, pulses and wholegrain bread and pasta as the basis for your eating plan.

Remember, A Few Pounds Could Be Enough!

If you're overweight, the good news is that to have a regular cycle you don't need to be stick thin. 'Sometimes just losing a few pounds can make a big difference to the way you ovulate,' says Professor Stephen Franks.

Don't Overdo The Exercise

Exercise is a must for optimum health and fertility, but taken to extremes it can cause periods to become irregular or even stop. Check with your doctor to see if your exercise routine is appropriate.

Tackle Emotional Eating

'I find it hard to get by without chocolate and sweets. I know they aren't good for me and they probably make my symptoms worse but they

make me feel better. I've tried cutting down but sometimes I feel so low only a bar of chocolate will do.' MANDY, 24

Losing weight can be a difficult issue, especially if you have PCOS. But if you're struggling to stick to a healthy eating regime to boost your fertility, it's time to look at your relationship with food. After all, until you sort this out, you're making it extra hard for yourself to stick to any new diet plan.

So, do you comfort eat with foods that you know aren't good for you?

Many women have a complex relationship with food and comfort eat in response to stress or difficult and painful emotions. With PCOS the problem can intensify owing to the moods swings and sugar cravings often linked with the condition. There are also the body image insecurities and weight management problems that become a part of it. So if you want to change to a healthy eating plan, it is crucial that you first heal your emotional relationship with food — you're setting yourself up for struggling and feelings of failure if you don't.

If you know you always reach for the cake or chocolate when you're blue or stressed, your first step to improved fertility through good nutrition isn't to focus on what you are eating, but to understand your relationship with food so that you can move towards a more healthy attitude and free yourself from emotional eating. Once you do this, you can eat what is good for you without feeling deprived and enjoy the occasional treat without feeling guilty. Whether you need to deal with stress, depression, getting mood swings under control or building your self-esteem and body image, you need to stop these issues sabotaging your weight loss plan. (To find the right support, information and advice, see our Resource Guide on page 275.)

GET MEDICAL HELP

If weight loss is proving frustrating and you know it will really help improve your chances of conception, you don't have to struggle alone. Talk to your doctor about referring you to a dietician or nutritionist who can work out a specific diet plan for you and help you stick to it.

Drug-Assisted Weight Loss

If you have a lot of weight to lose, there are more serious measures that your doctor can discuss with you, such as weight loss drugs like Reductil. Reductil is an appetite suppressant – basically it makes you feel satisfied with less food. Women with PCOS can lose weight on Reductil but there can be unpleasant side effects, which include nausea, headaches and a nasty taste in the mouth. Also, if you aren't eating that much already Reductil isn't ideal. The drug is not recommended if you are pregnant or trying to have a baby.

Another option is a new slimming pill, which is thought to be able to help people quit smoking and slim down at the same time. The drug, Rimonabant, works by blocking the circuits in the brain that control the urge to eat and smoke. The makers, French firm Sanofi-Synthelabo, hope to market the drug in 2005. In one trial the drug helped people to shed an average of 9kg (20lbs) in a year. And in a second, it was found to double the chances of smokers successfully quitting – at least in the short term. Dr Robert Anthenelli of the University of Cincinnati, who directed the smoking study, said: 'We think this might be the ideal compound for people who are overweight and smoke.' It's important to point out though that, like Reductil, this pill may not be safe to take if you are pregnant or trying for a baby. As always, discuss with your doctor.

Your doctor can also look at ketosis, a method where you eat only high protein foods to encourage your body to break down fat. This is still a controversial method for women with PCOS as experts cannot agree on whether it is safe in the long term, but in the short term it can offer the benefits of fast weight loss for women who really need to lose a lot of weight. However, it must be done under medical supervision with regular monitoring.

There is also the option of bariatric surgery in cases where nothing else has worked, and your healthcare practitioner feels the benefits outweigh the risks. As with any surgery, you need to be advised throughout the assessment and process by your healthcare practitioner. 'Surgery can be valuable if your BMI is above 35, but in the UK, the NHS usually restricts this surgery until a person is much heavier,' says Professor Adam Balen. 'If you want to discuss this option, ask your healthcare practitioner about banding or bypass surgery – preferably laparoscopic if weight loss is not achievable by diet and exercise. However, it is essential to get nutritional advice and you should not try and conceive until your weight is stabilised.'

STUBBORN PROBLEM THREE: A STRESSED-OUT LIFESTYLE

Sometimes it's easier to take on diet plans and exercise routines than it is to look at the stressed-out whirl your life has become. And if it's been easier for you to make changes to what you eat and how much you exercise than to manage to unwind and ease your feelings of stress (which can mount up when you're trying for a baby, too), you need to focus on this area for a while – it's amazing how many women with PCOS we talked to found that even when they were doing everything else right, this one piece of the jigsaw wasn't fitting into place – but when it did, their periods came back and pregnancy often followed.

'It's worth investing in de-stressing your life,' says **NAOMI, 34,** *who has a son, Noah, aged three. 'I was so rigid in following a healthy diet and exercise plan, making sure I was doing well at work, staying in touch with my family and elderly parents, as well as trying to fit in romantic evenings with my husband in order to try and get in the mood for baby making, that I was wound up so tight. A friend of mine who didn't have PCOS but who had found it hard to get pregnant suggested I start going for massage, and having some chill out time, looking after myself instead of my career and my family for a change – and something just clicked. I started having massage, giving myself the time for long baths, reading books which I hadn't done in so long and turning down invitations out with friends and family just to have some time for me and for our relationship. Just four months later I got pregnant.'*

So how does stress have such a powerful effect on fertility – and why is it worth trying to reduce it if you have PCOS and are struggling to conceive? If you're under stress, too much prolactin is released and the normal messages between your brain (hypothalamus and pituitary) and ovaries can be affected, interfering with your ovaries' ability to give out the right balance of hormones.[184]

Invest in Some 'Me' Time

If the ideas in the seven-step plan aren't helping you to unwind very well, it's time to invest in a bigger commitment to 'me-time'.

As we suggested in the previous chapter, studies have shown how yoga and meditation can help ease tension. But yoga can do far more than that. Studies have shown that the deep breathing and stretching exercises of yoga can also help restore hormonal balance.[185] Meditation, like yoga, can also stimulate feelings of calm and tranquility and enhance your feelings of control.[186]

Try this mini-meditation to get you started:

Mini-Meditation

Find a place where you feel comfortable and imagine each part of your body relaxing. Begin with your scalp and work down to your toes while mentally repeating a neutral thought (try a colour or a cloudless sky). Concentrate on your breathing and when thoughts break through the calm, which they will, just let them come and go. After five minutes, open your eyes and sit quietly for a few moments before getting up and continuing your ordinary day.

Home Aromatherapy

Aromatherapy is a natural treatment that uses the therapeutic properties of essential oils, extracted from the flowers, leaves, stem barks or wood, of aromatic plants and trees. Essential oils can be extremely potent concentrates. They can be absorbed into the skin, hair and lungs, through massage, bathing and inhaling. Oils in the bloodstream will circulate for several hours, while those inhaled will stimulate the limbic system in the brain, which deals with emotions.

Recent research from Germany, Japan and Thailand is beginning to provide the scientific backing for this healing art. It has suggested jasmine essential oil is a powerful anti-depressant that relieves anxiety and lifts mood, and may work in the brain in a similar way to the drug valium.[187] It has also revealed the anti-inflammatory properties of rose, thyme and cloves[188]; as well as showing that linalool, a chemical component of lavender and lemon essential oils, can alter blood chemistry to reduce stress[189]; that ylang ylang reduces blood pressure and creates a calming effect when applied via the skin[190]; and rose essential oil applied via the skin also slows breathing rate and reduces blood pressure compared to a placebo, creating a relaxing effect.[191]

'Just remember smells are powerful, and so aromatherapy can be subjective as well as chemical,' says Jennie Harding, Product Technical Adviser for international aromatherapy company Tisserand and author of *The Essential Oils Handbook*. 'If you don't like a smell such as ylang ylang or patchouli, or even rose, you won't find a treatment with them uplifting or stress-relieving. If you do like a smell, the treatment will be enhanced.'

Aromatherapy Oils for Stress and Period Problems

Oils of particular relevance for helping soothe stress and restore irregular periods are: lavender, clary sage, geranium, jasmine, melissa, rose, sandalwood, neroli and ylang ylang.

Massage your abdomen, neck and shoulders as often as possible (or get a friend or partner to do it for you so you can totally relax!) with a total of two drops of your chosen oils in a teaspoon of carrier oil, such as sweet almond oil or pure sunflower oil; or soak in a warm bath laced with a total of four drops of essential oil in a teaspoon of carrier oil, or a tablespoon of full fat milk. You can also unwind to the scent of your favourite oil dropped on to a vaporizer or burner. Try and turn your aromatherapy treatment into a regular treat and really enjoy it.

If, after trying these routes to beat your stubborn PCOS problems, you still feel you need something more to help you on your way to conception, the next chapters are on natural and medical fertility treatments. If you have the time and inclination you could try the natural therapies first before moving on to medical intervention. Or you may decide with your healthcare provider that using the natural therapies alongside the orthodox ones is the best bet for you. Either way, the information you need to help you find your way is contained in the next two chapters of the book.

Chapter Four

· · · · · · · · · · ·

Fertility Treatments The Natural Way: Your Options with Complementary Therapies

As we've been seeing in the previous chapters, there's a lot you can do to help yourself in order to boost your fertility if you have PCOS. But this section of the book looks at what other people can do to help, too. If you feel it's the right time to try fertility treatments, the natural option of complementary therapies has a lot to offer, as long as you choose a reputable, well-qualified practitioner. Meanwhile, keep on going with your self-help programme as this will enhance the power of any therapies you use – the healthier you are, the quicker they can get to work. You may want to try the self-help/complementary therapy combination for a few months or longer, depending on what stage you're at in your journey. But you can also use them both alongside orthodox medical fertility treatments for a triple approach if that feels right.

WHAT DOES 'COMPLEMENTARY' MEAN?

'Complementary therapies' are so called because tentative research shows that they can be used effectively to complement, or support, mainstream treatment.[192] Philip Holm, chairman of Issue, the National Fertility Association of the UK, says, 'Due to increased coverage in the media of the alternative field, people are more open to trying more holistic methods to boost their fertility. Many of our members have used alternative therapies and believe they have been successful.'

Practitioners of alternative medicine also claim that they can help women with PCOS to conceive, but medical experts still differ wildly in their opinions.[193] You will need to discuss this with your healthcare practitioner, ideally seeking their support if you want to try this route, and using word of mouth recommendations to get a good practitioner who is happy to share information with you and your doctor so you can all work together.

Current PCOS research cannot give definitive statistics on what will work for who and for how long – as so little has been done to explore this avenue: 'It's a tricky one and more research is needed,' says Dr Simon Fishel, Director of the Centres for Assisted Reproduction (CARE) at Park Hospital in Nottingham, UK. 'But I have an open mind. Fertility seems to be affected by so many factors – lifestyle, stress, emotions and maybe alternative medicine is addressing these issues, so I do feel there is a place for it.'

But don't forget, the fact that these are natural therapies means you can go through conventional routes and use them to assist, enhance and support this treatment, too. Dr Sarah Temple (see Resource Guide on page 275) says, 'Complementary therapies are useful for rebalancing the body and making women feel ready for pregnancy. A lot of my patients have found acupuncture or reflexology helpful. If you do decide to have IVF, it's stressful. These women were glad they were also doing hypnotherapy, meditation or yoga to help them cope.'

That's not saying that alternative therapies don't have a physical effect on our bodies but, until more research is done, we won't know in scientific or medical terms what that effect is. But anecdotally, within the PCOS Internet unity, there is a growing feeling among women that many therapies do seem to work for them.

BE CAREFUL IN YOUR CHOICE

However, having problems trying to get pregnant can make you very vulnerable so you do need to make sure that you aren't being ripped off. 'Always choose someone who has been registered with the appropriate training organization,' says Nicky Wesson, author of Alternative Infertility Treatments. 'Find a therapy which feels right for you. Do your research and make an informed decision of what you feel may work for you. Find a therapist you like and trust and avoid anything which your intuition tells you is extreme or inappropriate.' She also suggests that you treat any therapist with caution who expects you to spend hundreds of pounds on products that can only be bought through them.

Make sure all your healthcare providers communicate well with you and with each other, and that you have been checked out medically so you know that PCOS definitely is the problem you need to tackle. And use as many email groups, support groups and PCOS contacts as you can to find out which natural therapy and practitioner seems right for you.

WHICH THERAPIES WORK WELL WITH PCOS?

Most complementary therapies look at you as a whole person, whose body and emotions, lifestyle and experience all play a part in creating the health problems you're experiencing. As the main root of the PCOS fertility problem is the underlying metabolic and hormonal imbalances, the natural approach taken by therapists from most disciplines will be to try and work on creating hormonal harmony, in order to bring regular periods, ovulation and the right conditions in your body and mind to encourage conception.

The therapy or therapies you choose will depend on what your problems are, which one you like the sound of, which one makes logical sense to you as an approach, and, perhaps, which one you hear recommended by friends or other women with PCOS in your local area, or via your local or internet support groups. Another good way to find a local well-qualified practitioner is to contact the associations governing national standards of practice and qualifications, who will list all their accredited practitioners for you (see our Resource Guide on page 275).

Although medical expert opinion is still divided, many women with PCOS who we have spoken to found the following natural therapies – when administered by a properly qualified therapist, ideally with a knowledge of PCOS or experience in treating PCOS patients – had profound results.

These therapies are the ones we found most women had used with positive results, and/or which have some research backing them up as valid options to explore if you have PCOS and need help with fertility. But remember – always seek the help of a qualified practitioner before trying these therapies as some remedies are not recommended for use during pregnancy.

Nutritional Therapy Plus Lifestyle Changes

Everything we've been telling you is really effective and you can do for yourself but a nutritional therapist can, on top of lifestyle changes and healthy eating, help you work out what specific nutrients you may be lacking, and help you work out a programme of diet and supplements uniquely tailored for you and your lifestyle.

Much of the advice given by a nutritional therapist will be the same as the advice given in the PCOS fertility-boosting action plan. You've seen how important preconceptual care is for boosting your chances and you've also seen how healthy lifestyle recommendations and certain supplements have scientific backing. For example, studies show that weight management can help women with PCOS conceive, certain nutrients such as B6 are linked to increased fertility and taking a daily multivitamin can not only help boost your fertility but can also help boost your chances with assisted conception, a Univeristy of Leeds study shows.[194] Of all the natural therapies you might like to explore, healthy diet and lifestyle changes are the most sensible and the most helpful.

Note: When taking any kind of supplement, always seek advice from a dietician, doctor or nutritional therapist before self-medicating.

Herbal Medicine

Along with nutritional therapy, acupuncture and reflexology, herbalism seems to be the most popular choice for women with PCOS, and has shown some very good results. Many women find it's a logical therapy, simply using the medicinal power of plants in their natural state to help boost health and wellbeing, as opposed to using synthesized extracts or isolated compounds as many drugs do (and so many of those drugs are based originally on plants anyway – for instance, aspirin is extracted from white willow bark; the heart drug digitalis comes from the foxglove; and the diabetes drug metformin, now used for PCOS, was inspired by a herb called goat's rue).

'Western medical herbalism can be extremely effective in balancing the hormones, increasing the function of the ovaries and helpful in improving the function of the pituitary gland, the master gland that controls the hormones in the body. Many women with irregular cycles have found herbs are excellent for balancing their hormones and therefore regulating their cycles and aiding conception,' says Julie Whitehouse, Senior Lecturer in Medical Herbs at the University of Westminster, London, UK.

A medical herbalist, according to Whitehouse, will take a full medical and personal history and look at your lifestyle, diet and environment. They will ask about any vitamins, minerals or drugs that you might be taking, and make any recommendations that might be necessary. They then might give you a combination of herbal tinctures to take several times a day and perhaps recommend that you delay trying to conceive for three months while your body is strengthened.

Chinese Herbs

Western medical herbalism differs from Chinese herbal medicine in the nature of the herbs involved, which may be grown in China and often used in conjunction with acupuncture. Zita West, a former NHS midwife and acupuncturist, uses a combination of Chinese herbs, nutritional therapy and acupuncture and reports great success in treating hormonal disturbances, including PCOS: 'The whole principle of Chinese medicine is that you need to be at maximum strength to conceive,' says West. There is more research evidence available regarding Chinese herbal medicine than there is for Western medical herbalism.[8]

Chinese herbs can help improve general health and readiness for conception and can be generally supportive during infertility treatment. For example, a study at the Department of Gynaecology, Second Affiliated Hospital, Hebei Medical College, Shijiazhuang, reported the treatment of cases with menstrual disorder.[195] The results showed that ovulatory rate was significantly higher in the group treated with traditional Chinese herbs and clomifene (see Glossary) than that of the group who were treated either with clomifene or with herbal treatment, showing that a combination of Western and Chinese herbal medicine may have advantages.

The following herbal treatments have all been used by women with PCOS who have fertility problems or irregular periods with varying degrees of success, and you may find these names come up if you visit a herbalist for a tailor-made prescription. Remember that these are powerful substances, and large amounts of any herb or dietary supplements should only be taken under the guidance of a doctor or a qualified consultant or herbalist, preferably one with experience of treating women with PCOS.

Herbal Treatments

Agnus Castus

Agnus castus (vitex/chasteberry tree) has been shown to stimulate and normalize the function of the pituitary gland, which in turn helps to balance hormone output from the ovaries and stimulate ovulation.[196] Agnus castus also keeps prolactin secretion in check in rats, and excessive prolactin can prevent ovulation. Vitex is used as a herbal treatment for infertility, particularly in cases with established luteal phase defect (shortened second half of the menstrual cycle) and high levels of the hormone prolactin. In one trial, 48 women (aged 23 to 39) who were diagnosed with infertility took vitex once daily for three months.[197–199] Seven women became pregnant during the trial, and 25 experienced normalized progesterone levels – which may increase the chances for pregnancy.

In another double-blind trial, significantly more infertile women became pregnant after taking a product whose main ingredient is vitex (the other ingredients were homeopathic preparations), than did those who took a placebo.[200] The amount used in this trial was 30 drops of fluid extract twice a day, for a total of 1.8 ml per day. This specific preparation is not available in the United States but there are many tinctures of vitex available in health stores or from medical herbalists.

Some doctors recommend taking 40 drops of a liquid extract of vitex each morning with water. Approximately 35–40 mg of encapsulated powdered vitex (one capsule taken in the morning) provides a similar amount. Vitex should be discontinued once a woman becomes pregnant.

Black Cohesh

Also known as black cohosh, this herb has a balancing effect on hormones and is often prescribed by medical herbalists for women with PCOS and irregular cycles.[201]

Dong Quai

A Chinese herb also called angelica which is well known as a tonic for the female reproductive system, regulating hormonal control and improving the rhythm of the menstrual cycle.[202]

Liquorice

A Japanese study has found that the liquorice plant herb helped women with PCOS and irregular periods, but the herb should only be taken under professional supervision as it can be taken only to help regulate your cycle and not when you are trying to get pregnant.

Sairei-to

The Chinese herbal medicine sairei-to may be a useful treatment for women with PCOS and irregular cycles according to research at the Department of Obstetrics and Gynaecology at Nippon Kokan Hospital in Kagawa, Japan.[203]

Shakuyaku-Kanzo-to (TJ-68)

A study in the *International Journal of Fertility* showed encouraging results when infertile women were treated with shakuyaku-kanzo-to.[204]

Shatawari

A popular Ayurvedic tonic used by some women to help normalize the hormonal imbalances of PCOS that cause irregular cycles.

Siberian Ginseng

Siberian ginseng is believed to help your body adapt to stress and balance blood sugar and is often recommended to women with PCOS and irregular cycles. It is not recommended, though, if you are trying to get pregnant as it can have potentially harmful implications for a developing baby.[205,h]

Unicorn Root

A North American herb said to be useful for women with delayed or absent periods. White peony is another herb, like unicorn root, that may help normalize the balance of hormones.

Unkei-to

When women with irregular periods were treated with the Japanese herb unkei-to in a controlled study, the rate of menstrual improvement for women with PCOS was 50 percent.[206]

Wild Yam

Wild yam is an anti-inflammatory agent with a weak hormonal activity in the body, which can improve menstrual function and fertility.

Herbs can also be a powerful force in balancing insulin levels and reducing insulin resistance in PCOS, according to Dr Ann Walker, medical herbalist and former Senior Lecturer in Human Nutrition at University of Reading. When treating many women with PCOS, as well as diabetic patients in conjunction with the local hospitals, Dr Walker often uses bilberry, goat's rue, cinnamon and fenugreek for people with insulin problems, as well as holy basil for more extreme cases.

Reflexology

Many women with PCOS have found reflexology helpful, saying that it relaxes them and helps their cycles become more regular. Reflexology feels like a vigorous foot massage, during which the reflexologist stimulates specific reflex points on your foot, which are thought to link into energy channels called meridians running throughout the body, as in Chinese Medicine and acupuncture. By pressuring one reflex point in the foot, the reflexologist influences the energy flow around all the other organs and body areas that run along that meridian.

'Reflexology is one of the most effective ways of rebalancing the entire endocrine system,' says UK-based reflexologist Jacqui Garnier (www. jacquigarnier.com), who has PCOS herself and who uses reflexology to help other women. 'It is particularly successful when used in conjunction with a healthy diet and lifestyle. As a balancing treatment, it has been known to have success rates as high as 88 percent in infertility; it can regulate cycles, tone the uterus, encourage ovulation and improve the function of the ovaries; it can balance heavy and painful periods and reduce the stress so often associated with coping with the symptoms of PCOS.'

There has been little research done on the efficacy of reflexology in infertility, although a small trial in Denmark examined 108 women with an average age of 30 who had been trying to conceive for an average of 6.7 years. Many dropped out of the trial, but 19 of the remaining 61 conceived within six months of completing the treatment.

Aromatherapy

Whilst there is little evidence to suggest that aromatherapy can directly help infertility, it can certainly help alleviate the emotional stresses associated with infertility and going through fertility treatment.

Work carried out by Dr Gary Schwartz, former Professor of Psychology and Psychiatry at Yale University, found that the aromas of some essential oils by themselves affect the nervous system and even reduce blood pressure. The scent of spice apple, for example, was found to reduce blood pressure by an average of three to five points in healthy volunteers. Infertility problems can create enormous emotional stresses and certainly aromatherapy is an excellent way to help counter such stress and induce relaxation. And, as we have seen, stress does in itself affect your hormones and insulin balance, and extreme stress can delay or even stop your periods.

Recent research has proved the calming, relaxing and anti-stress effects of essential oils and aromatherapy massage. Massage with jasmine essential oil was shown to be mood lifting and relaxing, in research from Thailand.[187] Linalool, a chemical component of lavender and lemon essential oils, has been shown to reduce stress levels by altering chemical components in the blood in Japanese research.[189] And two separate studies which compared ylang ylang and rose essential oils applied via the skin, to placebos, showed they both lowered blood pressure and induced a relaxing effect.[190,191]

UK aromatherapist and reflexologist Frances Box, who specializes in enhancing fertility, believes aromatherapy oils, do in themselves have something to offer in boosting fertility. After all, they are potent plant oils, which get into the bloodstream through the skin (like the medication in HRT or nicotine patches), and can have a chemical effect in the body. 'Rose is known as the queen of oils,' she says. 'It's traditionally used for infertility because it contains a substance similar to oestrogen.'

'Relaxation is a large part of the process,' she says, using oils such as lavender and ylang ylang and marjoram, which work at relaxing the nervous systems. Many of her clients have had or are having IVF and ideally she likes to carry out her therapies alongside it: 'IVF is very stressful, what with counting days, taking temperatures and samples and being on tenterhooks about the outcome. So my first role is to relax clients who are usually depressed, anxious and stressed to the hilt. When you're stressed, it doesn't just affect your mind but your hormones too. Prolactin, for example, is a hormone that is influenced by stress, which can affect a woman's fertility. I believe that if you reduce stress, you improve your chances of fertility.'

The therapeutic massage combined with selected essential oils certainly makes aromatherapy an excellent aid in countering the effects of stress and inducing relaxation. Massage improves the blood circulation in several ways without putting additional strain on the heart. It helps the flow of blood through the veins and also stimulates the nerves that control the blood vessels. It has the added benefit of relaxing tense muscles and tight connective tissues, which may have been constricting blood vessels, and thus enables blood to flow more freely. It is for this reason that soothing massage helps reduce emotional tension, induces relaxation and calms stress-related conditions. It will therefore help improve your general health and wellbeing.

Acupuncture

Acupuncture may be one of the best researched complementary therapies – many women with PCOS seem to have found it most helpful for kick-starting absent periods and regulating cycles. Some research has also shown that it can have a balancing effect on your hormones, which is particularly good for women with PCOS.[207,208] Research on the benefits of Chinese medicine for women with irregular periods has also produced encouraging results.[209] Traditional acupuncturists treat the whole person rather than a disease, and therefore attempt to get to the root cause of the problem rather than treating the symptoms and, like other holistic practitioners, will consider all lifestyle and environmental factors before commencing treatment.

'Acupuncture is based on the principle of influencing the flow of vital energy around the body using needles. It is deceptively simple, correcting imbalances to assist the body's own recuperative powers to restore harmony and vital function,' says Susan Birch, who has been an acupuncturist for 12 years, specializing in fertility for the last four. She has recently opened The Centre for Optimum Fertility, in France, where couples can go for a four-day residential stay in rural France, which aims to offer an environment of deep relaxation as clients undergo treatment.

'Acupuncture boosts fertility as it helps to invigorate the flow of blood and energy to the lower abdominal area. For women, it will assist in regulating the menstrual cycle, boost ovulation and improve fertility. I have had great success in treating endometriosis, blocked fallopian tubes, ovarian cysts and infertility-related hormonal imbalances, like PCOS,' she says.

There is recent published evidence to show acupuncture can help with PCOS specifically. Women with PCOS can see improvements in hormone levels and menstrual bleeding pattern with a mix of acupuncture and exercise, revealed research from the University of Gothenburg, Sweden.[210]

In the study, published in the *American Journal of Physiology-Endocrinology and Metabolism*, a group of women with PCOS were given acupuncture where the needles were stimulated both manually and with a weak electric current at a low frequency. A second group exercised at least three times a week (and a third group acted as controls).

'The study shows that both acupuncture and exercise reduce high levels of testosterone and lead to more regular menstruation,' says docent associate professor Elisabet Stener-Victorin, who is responsible for the study. 'Of the two treatments, the acupuncture proved more effective.' Another piece of research recently carried out at the University of Virginia, USA, suggests acupuncture can help increase the chances of pregnancy in PCOS. This is echoed by fertility expert Emma Cannon (www.emmacannon.co.uk), based in the UK, who works alongside gynaecologists and fertility specialist with Chinese Medicine, to help with fertility problems. 'With irregular cycles, I normally see a difference within 2 to 3 menstrual cycles,' she says.

There has also been a study indicating acupuncture could be used to successfully treat depression during pregnancy, a time when some women are advised to reduce their intake of anti-depressant medication.[211]

Hypnotherapy: The Mind/Body Connection

Hypnotherapy works on the premise that there are two states of consciousness – the conscious and the subconscious – which may be at odds with each other. 'I believe that while a woman might consciously want a baby, her subconscious may be stopping her from getting pregnant,' says Elizabeth Muir, a clinical psychologist based in London who specializes in helping women who have 'unexplained infertility'. 'Most of the women I see have psychosomatic infertility related to conflicts, or unresolved issues about having a baby. A combination of counselling and hypnotherapy can remove these problems,' she says. Muir also believes that, if women have psychological blocks towards having a baby, the body will manifest this resistance in conditions such as endometriosis or polycystic ovaries. Muir's clients range from ages 37 to 45 and she claims a 45 percent success rate, based on live births resulting from conceptions that took place within her 10 suggested sessions of treatment, or within one year since completion of treatment.

Julie Gerland is a clinical hypnotherapist and founder of the Center of Universal Unity in Hong Kong. She also specializes in emotional clearing which she believes is necessary for parenting. There is huge pressure on women these days to have the perfect life, body, job, partner and family, but you may have your doubts and insecurities about motherhood and feel pressurized to conceive by those around you. It's important to find out what you really want. 'Subconscious worries can prevent conception, so hypnotherapy can deal with doubts about your future role as a mother,' says Julie.

There was some evidence published in the European Journal of Clinical Hypnosis in 1994 that hypnotherapy could help in medically unexplained, functional and psychosomatic infertility. If you are interested in this route you may also like to try a hypnotherapy CD called Prepare to Conceive, which has been developed by Nourish, a natural fertility programme that encourages couples to improve their emotional and physical health before planning for a baby (see also the Resource Guide on page 275).

Homeopathy

'Homeopathy is a method of helping the body heal itself using very dilute substances – many derived from plants, which at higher doses would produce the symptoms being treated – we explain it by saying "like treats like",' says Annetta Kershaw, a qualified homeopath practising in Keighley in Yorkshire, UK. If you think of how vaccination works along the same principle it can help to explain the logic behind this system of medicine, which has had scientists puzzled as to how it actually brings about some very effective results.

Although Kershaw has much success in helping women conceive, she does not claim to 'specialize' in PCOS-related infertility because, by its very nature, homeopathy treats the whole person rather than the symptom. 'We would see infertility as simply a symptom and we would concentrate on looking at the imbalances of the whole person – emotional, physical and mental – which could be causing the infertility.

Therefore, there is no simple recipe to treat infertility because every individual is unique,' she says.

This is why homeopaths will take a detailed life and case history from every patient, and why a range of 'constitutional' remedies exist corresponding to different types of person. If a homeopath can find your constitutional remedy by working out what type of person you are – emotionally, physically and in the way you relate to the world around you – this is thought to help to unlock some of your basic underlying health problems. On top of this, there are many homeopathic remedies designed to relieve specific symptoms – anything from nausea to acne.

Homeopathic remedies assist your own system clear itself of any imbalance. Remedies are used to treat symptoms such as irregular menstrual cycles; some will target the uterus or ovaries and others will treat any mental or emotional imbalances that your therapist may think are holding you back from conceiving.

In a 2000 German study, 30 infertile women with hormonal problems were given homeopathic remedies, while a matched group was treated with placebo.[212] The results for the homeopathic group were encouraging and increasingly medical experts are suggesting homeopathy as a complement or alternative to conventional medicine.[213]

Chapter Five

Fertility Treatments The Medical Way: Getting The Best Medical Science Has to Offer

Hopefully, by the time you read this section of the book you will have a better understanding of how the complex and delicate balance of your hormones can be upset by your diet and lifestyle. But when you're trying to get pregnant and nothing happens, it's easy to panic, so in this section we'll tell you where and how to get help for fertility problems and the kind of fertility treatments most likely to be recommended to you if you have PCOS.

Being in a healthy state of mind and body will increase your chances of success with fertility treatment. The greatest chance of pregnancy will occur when your body is at maximum harmony – in hormonal balance. Follow the advice in our preconception plan, take care of yourself, live well and, above all, live happy.

The first step to successfully manage your fertility treatment is to find a good doctor. You need to find a fertility specialist – someone who treats women and couples with fertility problems and who, ideally, has experience of treating women with PCOS.

THE COST OF INFERTILITY

'Having a baby is the most important thing in my life right now. It's already cost us more than we can afford but however much it costs I'm going to make it happen.' Toni, 39

'When I saw the cost of treatment I was shocked. I'm a nurse and my partner is unemployed. We can't put our hands on money like that. Right now I just don't know what I'm going to do. I do sometimes wonder, though, if this just isn't meant to be.' Elizabeth, 26

Infertility is now big business in both Britain and America. About 85 percent of fertility treatments are carried out by private clinics. If you have PCOS and want to have a baby, you can feel very vulnerable and could end up spending a great deal of money to find out why, and then buy treatment. The average cost of a single IVF treatment in the UK is close to £3,000 and in the US $5,000.

In the UK you can, of course, go on the NHS waiting list. In February 2004 the government announced that infertile women under 40 will get free IVF treatment on the NHS – but only one attempt. Health Secretary John Reid said he wanted to end the postcode lottery, where free IVF depends on where you live. This is a great start, but internationally respected gynaecologist Professor Robert Winston, who specializes in fertility, believes that offering couples just one attempt isn't enough, as it often takes two or more attempts to get pregnant. So if your first attempt at IVF fails and you want to try again, much will depend on the rationing of resources for fertility treatment in the area where you live, your age – in some areas women over 35 will be refused further treatment – and your circumstances – some trusts make marriage or a stable relationship a condition. And your chances may also be reduced if you already have children or are a stepmother. 'It is utterly deplorable that a woman in her fifties can get help if she has money,' says Sheena Young of the National Infertility Awareness Campaign (NIAC), 'while a woman of 35 without the wherewithal may be condemned to no more help at all.' She sees budgets rather than bias as the problem. 'The denial of help is always about lack of money.'

Long waiting lists aren't good news if you have PCOS and time isn't on your side. So what can you do if waiting and remortgaging your home isn't an option? Fortunately, many women with PCOS won't actually need the more advanced and expensive treatments, like IVF. Preliminary testing and ovulation-boosting drugs, like Clomid, may be all that is needed and most tests and ovulation-boosting drugs can be provided and prescribed at a private fertility clinic. And if this is the case the cost would be more affordable, in the hundreds rather than the thousands.

FINDING A FERTILITY SPECIALIST

Unfortunately some fertility clinics are more ethical and honest with their clients than others, so it is worth taking the time to choose one you feel comfortable with. If you decide to be a paying client, rather than a patient at a state run clinic, you do have more control and have the opportunity to select an environment you feel happy in. Some clinics are small and friendly and you see the same doctor each time, whereas others are big hospital-based units.

When choosing a clinic try to find out about their success rates. Shop around. Ring up and ask for several brochures. Contact an infertility organization, such as CHILD in the UK, or RESOLVE in the US, for advice about choosing a clinic. If you live in the UK the Human Fertilisation and Embryology Authority (HFEA) is the licensing authority for infertility clinics and it produces league tables to show how successful they are.

Check your country's equivalent. You could also ask your family doctor to recommend a clinic or ask other women with PCOS via support groups. Choose three or four clinics that you like the sound of and which aren't too far away, and visit them or ask to speak to a senior consultant on the phone.

Questions To Ask When Deciding on a Clinic

- Are the consultants fully qualified?

- Will my specialist be an OB/GYN who has chosen additional training in reproductive endocrinology?

- Do the consultants have experience treating women with PCOS?

- What treatment and tests do they offer?

- Do they have any age restrictions?

- Do they have a waiting list?

- How successful are they in treating women with PCOS?

- Are there any 'hidden' costs?

- Do they offer a 24-hour, 7-day-a-week service so that I can be seen right away if need be?

- Will I be closely monitored when taking fertility drugs?

- What are their success rates in 'take home' live births?

- What are the costs?

- What might be covered by insurance?

Try to meet the specialist who will be in charge of your treatment before you make your final choice. Do you feel comfortable with them? Do they inspire you with confidence? What does your partner think?

Although clinics are supposed to report accurate success rates, this may not always be the case, especially in the US where the fertility industry thrives at $2 billion a year. If you are thinking of registering at any fertility clinic, never sign up immediately. Take your time, do your research, ask to speak to former patients, find out about the doctors treating you, contact advisory boards and seek a second, third and fourth opinion. This is a huge decision and it's vital that you feel comfortable with it.

How to Get the Most from Your Doctor

If your doctor recommends taking fertility drugs and there's a full waiting room outside and he or she clearly hasn't got the time to discuss PCOS at length, you may feel under pressure to make major decisions after a quick conversation. If that's the case don't be intimidated. Write down what you need to ask beforehand. Take notes and maybe bring a friend who can prompt you. If you feel you need more time, don't be afraid to ask the receptionist for a double appointment, or to book you in during your doctor's quietest time.

If you are concerned about the advice you've been given, there is nothing wrong with asking for a second opinion. Remember, it is your doctor's responsibility to provide all the information you need, and you should never feel obliged to commit to a decision on the spot – go away and get in touch with your PCOS support group to help you find more information. If the worst happens and your doctor is dismissive or rude about your concerns, try to remain calm and assertive – the assertive patient gets better care so be reasonable but firm. If you just don't get on with your doctor or fertility specialist, you can stay registered with the same surgery or clinic but ask to see another doctor when you book an appointment. You can also change surgeries or clinics altogether. If you are not happy with the care you receive, tell someone, such as another doctor, about the cause of your concern. Alternatively, ask about the procedures for complaints or contact your local Patient Advice and Liaison services for help.

The way to secure the best care for yourself is to take control. Learn to stand up for yourself in consultations and give yourself all the time and space you need to make one of the most important decisions of your life.

METHODS TO MONITOR OVULATION

To achieve pregnancy you need to know when and if you are ovulating and the most reliable way to determine this is to undergo a series of diagnostic tests. These tests are usually done in conjunction with noting cervical mucus or taking your temperature (see page 35 in Chapter Two).

Transvaginal ultrasound is an important tool for diagnosing PCOS and to determine if you're ovulating. This method uses sound waves to produce images of your reproductive organs. In this procedure the doctor inserts a hand-held cylinder-shaped instrument called a transducer into your vagina to measure your ovaries and check the uterine lining. The doctor can examine the size of your ovaries to see exactly how many follicles are developing and how big they are. To be considered the optimum size for conception, follicles should measure about 16–22 mm in diameter, and the uterine lining should be about 10–12 mm thick to sustain a pregnancy.

If you aren't having periods you may be given some progesterone or progestins to induce a bleed, and 21 days later (or, if your periods are regular, seven days after you think you may have ovulated), you may also be given a progesterone test. This test will tell you if an egg was released from the ovary. If it was released, your progesterone level should be significantly higher. If levels are low the chances are the egg was not released.

Some doctors suggest that you have an ultrasound, a progesterone test and a post-coital test, which is a bit like a pap test taken a few hours after sex to see if your partner's sperm is surviving in your cervical mucus. If you did ovulate successfully, your period will begin 14 days after ovulation, and if it doesn't you could already be pregnant!

If you didn't ovulate, your doctor may suggest that you try another progestin cycle or he or she may suggest fertility medication to induce ovulation.

Fertility Treatments to Induce Ovulation in Women With PCOS

Most of the drugs used to induce ovulation have unpleasant side effects, ranging from nausea to mood swings and insomnia, so make sure you ask your specialist to keep you fully informed. Bear in mind, too, that some studies indicate that fertility medication to induce ovulation may be associated with ovarian cancer and ovarian hyperstimulation syndrome – a rare but serious condition when the ovaries enlarge as a result of fertility treatment and which can cause damage not just to future fertility but to other organs.[214] 'It is common to have an exaggerated response to ovarian stimulation with PCOS,' says PCOS expert Dr Sam Thatcher. 'So if you've got PCOS you need to be aware that your chances of ovarian hyperstimulation may increase because there are already lots of partially developed follicles on your ovary, all in suspended animation, and fertility drugs are more likely to stimulate multiple follicles.'

PROCEED WITH CAUTION

There are still glaring gaps in our knowledge about the danger that fertility drugs may pose and whether the benefits outweigh the risks. Clinical trials haven't been done to establish links between several rounds of commonly prescribed fertility drugs, like Clomid, and ovarian cancer, but many experts believe there to be a link. In 2003 the journal Fertility and Sterility published a National Institutes of Health study showing that women who had taken Pergonal-type drugs had a risk of breast cancer two to three times greater than those who hadn't. Cancer, however, is not the only threat hanging over fertility drugs; they also carry the risk of anxiety, depression and chronic physical distress, such as chest pain, hives and severe, unexplained pain.

Many questions remained unanswered about the use and side effects of fertility drugs. Perhaps the answers will come one day but for now bear in mind that their use is still experimental and you should proceed with extreme caution. For all the promise that reproductive medicine can bring, it also breaks many hearts and bears risks that are as yet unknown.

FERTILITY DRUGS

The major benefit of taking fertility medication is that you have a better chance of ovulating and getting pregnant. These drugs work by stimulating egg production, encouraging ovulation, or by stabilizing hormone levels which could be inhibiting ovulation. A number of women with PCOS find that ovulation-inducing drugs work, but not every medication works for everyone.

'We'd been trying for four years to get pregnant and now that my thirtieth birthday was approaching I decided it was time to see a doctor.

All I had ever wanted was to be a mother. Even as a little girl I used to rock my little sister and sing her to sleep. I was the most sought after babysitter with my friends, but now I wanted to have a baby myself. I was diagnosed with PCOS and put on a course of Clomid therapy with a series of ultrasounds to determine the growth and size of my follicle. When it was large enough (a whopping 24 mm!) the doctor injected me in the hips, explaining that I needed this to help the egg release from its follicle. That injection really hurt and for a few days after I was sore. I expected the treatment to take a while and wasn't looking forward to another injection so you can imagine our shock when the pregnancy test turned positive.' ELIZABETH, 32

'I'd heard so much about how wonderful Clomid can be for women with PCOS and my sister, who's also got PCOS, got pregnant on her second cycle of Clomid, so I started my fertility treatment with high hopes. But when the fourth cycle failed I realized that Clomid wasn't going to be a miracle worker for me. My doctor suggested a final course of Clomid but this time with metformin too. It worked. I'm the proud mother of a baby boy, age three. Four months ago I had another course of Clomid with metformin and found out that I'm pregnant again – with twins. I couldn't be happier!' SONIA, 36

Complementary therapies which can help encourage regular ovulation and which can be used alongside fertility treatments to maximize your chances of success include acupuncture, reflexology, herbalism, hypnotherapy and relaxation techniques (see Chapter 4).[215] Do make sure, though, that you work with a qualified practitioner and that you tell your fertility specialist what you are doing, in order to check for any contraindications.

Male fertility test helps decide which treatment is best

A groundbreaking new test for male infertility, which will save time, money and heartache for couples around the world, has been developed at Queen's University Belfast. The medical breakthrough, known as the SpermComet, has resulted from more than a decade's research by Professor Sheena Lewis, who leads the Reproductive Medicine research group at Queen's.

The SpermComet provides unique information that no other test offers. By measuring damaged DNA in individual sperm, it can predict the success of infertility treatments and fast-track couples to the treatment most likely to succeed, leading to significantly reduced waiting times and improved chances of conception. As at June 2011 this is available at clinics in Glasgow, Scotland, and Dublin and Galway in the Republic of Ireland, but is planned to expand its reach over the coming years.

Clomifene Citrate (brand names Clomid and Serophone)

'Clomid is usually the first line therapy for induction of ovulation in PCOS,' says PCOS expert Dr Thatcher. It works by causing the body to produce more follicle-stimulating hormone and luteinizing hormones that promote egg growth. Once the brain senses increased oestrogen levels, it signals the LH surge that results in ovulation. '7 out of 10 women will ovulate with Clomid and around half of that number will get pregnant,' says Professor Bill Ledger, Professor of Obstetrics & Gynaecology at Sheffield University. 'These drugs are much cheaper than IVF and allow a much more normal conception, involving happy sex rather than medical practice. The best candidates for clomifene have a BMI of less than 30, or at the very most 35 (complications in pregnancy are greater in overweight women), and are under the age of 40. For women over

40 years, IVF is usually advised. Ideally you should have undergone pre-counselling so you understand the pros and cons of treatment, and what Clomid can realistically achieve.'

It can take a few cycles on Clomid to determine the right dosage for you, but the drug should not be taken for more than six months at a time. There are several potential side effects including headaches, depression, fatigue and a 5 to 10 percent risk of twins or triplets, as Clomid increases the number of preovulatory follicles and ovulations and therefore the chance of multiple pregnancy. 'Pre-treatment counselling should include discussion of the possibility of multiple births,' says Professor Ledger. 'A simple ultrasound scan can identify those women at risk of a multiple conception.'

More serious side effects include ovarian enlargement or hyperstimulation. If there are any changes in your vision or severe headaches when taking Clomid, tell your doctor immediately. Clomid can also have a negative impact on fertility by causing your cervical mucus to become hostile to sperm.

Because of the potential side effects your specialist will recommend you use the lowest dose of Clomid that results in ovulation. The usual starting dose is 50 mg (one tablet). Success is usually achieved at doses over 150 mg (three tablets a day), but the 'more is better' rule does not apply because higher doses can prevent rather than promote pregnancy. The dose needs to be adjusted according to body weight, with heavier patients needing more. Clomid may be started on day two, three, four or five of your cycle and is usually given over five days. A recent conference in San Diego looked at different ways to give Clomid to women with PCOS but concluded that there is no one regimen that is superior to the other.

If you haven't got pregnant after five or six cycles of Clomid, clearly the treatment isn't working. Research suggests that about two-thirds of women taking Clomid ovulate within four cycles and some studies show that about 35 percent achieve pregnancy.[216] If your doctor continues to recommend it, it might be wise to seek another opinion. Clomid treatment is fairly inexpensive, costing around £80 or $120 a treatment cycle. Studies also show that there is an increased risk of ovarian cancer with 12 or more cycles of Clomid, and women with PCOS must be followed with particular care.[217] Most doctors are unwilling to prescribe more than six cycles of Clomid at any one time, but every case needs to be discussed with your doctor or a fertility specialist to ensure the right decision is made in your case.

Insulin sensitizers

There are no specified contraindications for Clomid, and therefore taking metformin has not been proven to hinder the progress of Clomid. For a while it has been thought that taking both metformin and Clomid at the same time would provide the best environment for anovulatory treatment, but recent trials have indicated that Clomid alone is the most effective method.[218] The Royal College of Obstetricians and Gynaecologists, The American Society for Reproductive Medicine, and the European Society for Human Reproduction and Embryology are all sceptical of the use of metformin for fertility treatment, particularly in cases where the woman does not suffer from insulin sensitivity. A recent study from The Penn State College of Medicine proved the point: 'Our results show that you can't use ovulation as a surrogate for pregnancy,' said lead investigator Richard. S. Legro, MD, of the Department of Obstetrics and Gynecology. 'An ovulation on clomiphene treatment is twice as likely to result in pregnancy as an ovulation on metformin, thus all ovulations are not alike.' If you are insulin resistant or have diabetes, metformin may be beneficial. You need to discuss the use of metformin and Clomid with your specialist.

A word on safety for the baby – nearly 50 years of experience with this drug has shown that the rate of birth defects is not higher than that of the general population.

Gonadotrophin (HCG)

Gonadotrophins are drugs that stimulate your ovaries to release eggs by supplying your body with an extra amount of FSH or LH – the hormones that start egg production. Possible side effects include bloating, nausea, depression and hot flushes. There is also an increased risk of ovarian hyperstimulation (around 1 percent) and multiple pregnancy (around 20 percent).

With new information available, authors of a Cochrane Systematic Review have revised their conclusions about the relative effectiveness of two different treatments used to help women become pregnant. They now conclude that giving women gonadotrophin-releasing hormone (GnRH) antagonists (such as hCG, see below) leads to similar live-birth rates compared with GnRH agonists.[219] Previously they had concluded that women who used antagonists tended to have lower birth-rates than those using agonists.

In 2006, when the researchers reached their earlier conclusion, they were only able to draw data from 27 trials. Since then more research has been published, allowing them to consider the findings of 45 randomised controlled studies that involved a total of 7,511 women. 'This increased amount of data lets us get a much better idea of how well the two approaches compare,' says Dr Hesham Al-Inany, who was lead author of the research and works at Cairo University, Egypt. Dr Al-Inany led a multi-centre team, with researchers also based in the Netherlands and Canada. 'The reduction in ovarian hyperstimulation combined with a comparable live-birth rate mean justifies a move away from the standard GnRH agonist to using GnRH antagonists,' says Dr Al-Inany.

If this research is taken up by fertility experts, you may find a slightly different treatment programme is recommended to you.

The most common gonadotrophins are FSH, human menopausal gonadotrophin (hMG) and human chorionic gonadotrophin (hCG).

FSH
FSH (the follicle-stimulating hormone) controls ovulation, in partnership with LH. Because women with PCOS often have an elevated LH level, sometimes pure FSH is given to balance out the LH to FSH ratio. Once there are adequate levels of oestrogen and the follicle develops, an hCG shot is given to release the egg. There are different types of FSH available, but the most often prescribed are Fertinex, Gonal F and Follistim. FSH is given by daily injection and is usually expensive. Side effects can include mood swings and ovarian hyperstimulation.

Human Menopausal Gonadotrophin (hMG)
More commonly known as Pergonal and Repronex, this medication is an extract from the urine of menopausal women and contains LH and FSH which stimulate ovulation. It is given by injection, usually in the thigh or buttocks. Some research suggests that about 90 percent of women ovulate using hMG but only 60 percent conceive. Side effects can be mood swings and there is an increased risk of ovarian hyperstimulation, if not monitored properly, along with multiple pregnancy.

Human Chorionic Gonadotrophin (hCG)
It is this hormone that makes an ovary release its dominant follicle (the one that is ripest), and also helps keep your womb lining in place if you get pregnant. The drug hCG is used with other fertility medications including Clomid, FSH and hMG, to promote ovulation by triggering the LH surge. There is an increased risk of ovarian hyperstimulation and cyst

formation. In some women with PCOS a follicle develops well with other fertility medications but the egg is never released. If this is the case and the follicle appears ripe but LH fails to trigger release, your doctor can give you an injection of hCG to cause ovulation.

OVARIAN SURGERY

This is only an option if other medications have failed. There are two types of ovarian surgery – ovarian drilling, also known as diathermy, and wedge resection. Surgery can't cure PCOS but it can promote ovulation to increase your chances of pregnancy.

Ovarian drilling is an outpatient laparoscopic procedure where a laser is used to pierce the thickened coat of the ovary. The surgeon uses the laser to penetrate the cysts on each ovary. Fluid is drained from the ovary, eliminating many of the cysts. In turn the amount of testosterone produced is lowered, causing a decrease in LH. About 80 percent of women undergoing the procedure will ovulate and about 30–40 percent will get pregnant. Being close to your ideal weight will improve your chances of success. Possible risks include the normal risks of surgery along with possible adhesions and destruction of the ovary. Don't worry if you've had diathermy and it hasn't been successful – if the procedure was a success and recovery sound, you do still have the option of fertility drug treatment afterwards.

Wedge resection is a major procedure rarely performed today. It involves the surgical removal of cysts. It can increase the chances of ovulation but it carries with it a high risk of adhesions that can prevent pregnancy.

ASSISTED REPRODUCTIVE TECHNOLOGIES

'When every other option failed my doctor suggested IVF. I had no idea
what to expect and in retrospect it's probably a good thing I didn't. First
there were the injectable drugs to stimulate my ovary. They hurt and
made me feel sick. I had countless scans and blood tests to determine
if my eggs were big enough and to see if my hormone levels were right.
Then there was one last injection to help me ovulate. Exactly 36 hours
after that I had what is known as a follicle aspiration, where a needle is
passed through the vaginal wall, and with the use of ultrasound, fluid is
removed from the follicles by suction. Immediately after aspiration the egg
is isolated from the follicular fluid and placed along with my husband's
sperm in an incubator in a culture dish. I'm a bit of a coward when it
comes to needles and things so I opted for a general anaesthesia as I've
heard that all this can be quite painful.

About 48 hours later, the egg and sperm had formed an embryo
which was placed in my womb. I wanted general anaesthesia again for
implantation but my doctor reassured me that this wasn't necessary and
he was right. I didn't feel a thing. Then came the hardest part of all – the
waiting. For two weeks I was a prisoner in my home. My doctor had told
me to carry on with my life as normal but I couldn't. I didn't want to do
anything that might harm my baby. When the phone call came saying
it hadn't worked my world collapsed, but I immediately signed up for a
second round of treatment. That didn't work either. On my third round I
began to wonder if this was ever going to work and John and I started
to consider adoption. After the third implantation I went about my life as
normal, convinced that I wasn't pregnant. Then the phone rang. I went
into shock. We had done it. I was pregnant.' JANE, 37

Some women with PCOS who are not successful at getting pregnant using the treatments described earlier turn to assisted reproductive technology, or ART. These procedures can be extremely expensive and carry with them the risk of multiple births, ovarian hyperstimulation and high rates of miscarriage.[220] As always with fertility treatments, the advice is to proceed with extreme caution. Success rates are variable and depend on many factors: age; other problems, such as your partner's sperm quality and quantity; how experienced your doctor is; the quality of your eggs and the number of cycles attempted. Although many pregnancies with techniques like IVF and GIFT do occur on the first cycle, chances of pregnancy appear to be equal with each try through the first four attempts, and the average couple will undergo two or three attempts before a successful pregnancy. Although there are always exceptions, the pregnancy rate starts to decline after the fourth attempt and it is reasonable to review your options with your doctor and think about stopping after that.

Some reassuring news from the latest research is that whether you get pregnant in the traditional way or through assisted reproduction, it will have no effect on the birthing process or the baby. Researchers at the Norwegian University of Science and Technology looked at 1.2 million women's pregnancies between 1984 and 2006, with 8,229 of these pregnancies resulting from assisted reproduction technology. There was no reported difference in the birth weight, gestational age and preterm delivery of any of the babies. So what are your options?

Research has suggested that women with PCOS tend to produce many eggs but have lower fertilization rates with ART. 'Certainly we know,' says PCOS expert Dr Samuel Thatcher, 'that eggs from women with PCOS are not always "good." There is evidence to suggest that eggs extracted from the small cysts of PCOS ovaries have much less capacity to undergo development than do eggs from follicles of similar size in women without PCOS.'[222] So if you are thinking about ART you should consult your doctor or fertility specialist for an evaluation to assess your chances of success. Here are some of the techniques that might be discussed:

IVF (In Vitro Fertilization)

In this technique the woman's eggs are fertilized with her partner's sperm in a lab, and the resulting very young embryos are placed back into the womb so they can implant in the lining there. Sometimes, if several IVF attempts have been made, this is combined with 'assisted hatching', in which a tiny hole is made using a needle or chemical in the embryo's casing so it can attach itself more easily to the womb lining. The transfer takes only a few minutes and involves placing a small plastic tube through the cervix into the uterine cavity. No anaesthesia is required and usually minimal or no discomfort is felt.

The latest good news for IVF

- *Acupuncture could increase IVF success – whether it's real or not!* A review of seven clinical trials of acupuncture given with embryo transfer in women undergoing IVF suggests that acupuncture may improve rates of pregnancy. The studies encompassed data on over 1,366 women and compared acupuncture, given within one day of embryo transfer, with sham acupuncture, or no additional treatment. The reviewers found that acupuncture given as a complement to IVF increased the odds of achieving pregnancy. According to the researchers, the results indicate that 10 women undergoing IVF would need to be treated with acupuncture to bring about one additional pregnancy. The results, considered preliminary, point to a potential complementary treatment that may improve the success of IVF and the need to conduct additional clinical trials to confirm these findings.

A study comparing the effects of real and placebo acupuncture on pregnancy rates during assisted reproduction has found that, surprisingly, placebo acupuncture was associated with a significantly higher overall pregnancy rate than real acupuncture. The study, published online in the journal *Human Reproduction*, looked at real and placebo acupuncture given on the day of embryo transfer in 370 patients in a randomised, double blind trial (where neither the patients nor the doctors knew which treatment was being given). The researchers found that the overall pregnancy rate (defined by a positive urinary pregnancy test) for placebo acupuncture was 55.1%, versus 43.8% for the real acupuncture. One explanation is that 'sham' acupuncture is hard to create, and acupressure may be effective anyway.

- *Having IVF in spring might boost chances.* The success of an assisted reproduction procedure may depend on the season. This is the finding of new work presented at the World Congress of Fertility and Sterility, in Munich, Germany. All patients came from a single fertility center, the Assisted Fertilization Center in Sao Paulo, Brazil. Researchers looked at 435 patients in winter (representing 22.5% of the total sample), 444 in spring (23.0%), 469 in summer (24.2%), and 584 in autumn (30.3%). They found that the percentage of developing eggs (MII oocytes), high-quality embryos, implantation and pregnancy rates did not differ among the groups. Nevertheless the fertilization rate was significantly higher during the spring than during any other season (winter: 67.9; spring: 73.5%, summer: 68.7% and autumn: 69.0%). Lead author Dr Daniela Braga said, 'This work shows that IVF cycles may have a better outcome during the Spring. Our results show a significant difference in spring fertilization rate, with the fertilization rate in the spring being almost one and a half-times that of other seasons. In practical terms this may mean that if you are having real difficulty in conceiving, it may be better to have an assisted reproduction cycle during this season.'

- *Stress won't stop IVF working – but you increase your chances if you reduce it.* In a review of research published February 2011, fourteen studies with 3,583 infertile women undergoing a cycle of fertility treatment were included. The women were assessed before fertility treatment for anxiety and stress. The results show that emotional distress was not associated with whether or not a woman became pregnant. 'These findings should reassure women that emotional distress caused by fertility problems or other life events co-occurring with treatment will not compromise their chance of becoming pregnant,' says lead author Professor Jacky Boivin from the Cardiff Fertility Studies Research Group.

    But if you know you're stressed and want to do something about it, that can help too. 52 percent of the women participating in a Mind/Body Program for Infertility became pregnant compared with 20 percent of the control group participants, found a study published in June 2011, in Fertility and Sterility, a publication of the American Society of Reproductive Medicine. 'Intervening with mind body therapies is strongly indicated to help improve ivf outcomes,' said principal investigator Alice Domar, Ph.D, OB/GYN, Beth Israel Deaconess Medical Center and Executive Director of the Domar Center for Mind/Body Health at Boston IVF.

- *15 eggs increases risk of live birth.* An analysis of over 400,000 IVF cycles in the UK has shown that doctors should aim to retrieve around 15 eggs from a woman's ovaries in a single cycle in order to have the best chance of achieving a live birth after assisted reproduction technology. The study found a strong relationship between live birth rates and the number of eggs retrieved in one cycle. The live birth rate rose with an increasing number of eggs up to about 15; it levelled off between 15 and 20 eggs, and then steadily declined beyond 20 eggs.

Dr Coomarasamy, a Clinical Reader and Consultant in Reproductive Medicine and Surgery at the University of Birmingham (UK), and his colleagues analysed data from the UK's Human Fertilisation and Embryology Authority (HFEA) on 400,135 IVF cycles that took place anywhere in the UK between April 1991 and June 2008. 'Mild stimulation protocols aim to retrieve less than six to eight eggs; a standard stimulation should aim for 10-15 eggs, and we believe this is what is associated with the best IVF outcomes; when the egg number exceeds 20, the risk of OHSS becomes high,' said Dr Coomarasamy.

- *IVF chances increase if embryos rocked?* Scientists have discovered that if you rock embryos gently during the IVF process, pregnancy rates improve. So far, the experiments have only been done on mice, but the results are promising. When embryos are fertilised in the body in the normal way, they move all the time for the first day or two as they go down the fallopian tube and into the womb where they implant. During IVF, the eggs are left in a dish in an incubator and don't move at all. So, the team at the University of Michigan invented a device to gently rock embryos during IVF, and it increased pregnancy rates by 22% in mice. They believe it worked because the embryos that were gently rocked felt more at home. Trials in humans have now begun.

- *Could metformin make IVF safer?* 'There is some evidence that adding metformin to ovulation induction in women with PCOS undergoing IVF treatment reduces the risk of developing OHSS,' says Professor Adam Balen. Speak to your specialist about your options.

GIFT (Gamete-fallopian Transfer)

Although very popular in the 80s and 90s, GIFT is now used much less frequently than IVF. In this procedure the eggs are taken from the ovary, then sperm and eggs are simultaneously placed into the fallopian tubes, the tube through which the egg travels from the ovary to the uterus.

ZIFT (Zygote Interfallopian Transfer)

ZIFT involves the removal of eggs from the ovary, which are fertilized with sperm in the lab. A day later the embryos are placed into the fallopian tube.

IUI (Intrauterine Insemination)

Egg production is stimulated through the use of fertility medications and monitored closely by the doctor. When ovulation occurs, sperm is deposited directly into the uterus to shorten the distance to the ovary.

Intracytoplasmic Sperm Injection

A single sperm is injected into an egg through a very tiny needle in this procedure. Two days later, the resulting embryo is transferred into the uterus.

Donor Eggs

Here the mother-to-be receives eggs from another woman. The eggs are fertilized in the lab with the sperm from a partner or donor. Once fertilized, the eggs are placed into the uterus. Although the woman is not the genetic mother, she will be the birth mother.

HELPING YOURSELF

Adam Balen, Consultant Gynaecologist and Obstetrician and specialist in Reproductive Medicine and Surgery at Leeds General Infirmary, UK, is a great believer in individualism when it comes to fertility treatment for PCOS. 'Some treatments, like Clomid, help women with PCOS get pregnant, but PCOS is a complex disorder and there isn't one fertility treatment or approach per se. You have to treat each patient with PCOS as a unique individual to find what works best for her. Much will depend on body weight,' he says. 'These days we should start with metformin and then add in fertility drugs, like Clomid, if ovulation isn't happening.'

PCOS is complex and finding the right treatment for you will take time and patience but one thing remains certain – whatever treatment you are trying, you can help yourself. As we've seen, research has shown that even a basic multivitamin and mineral during fertility treatment can improve your chances of success with IVF. Fertility treatments can leave you feeling quite powerless but healthy diet and lifestyle changes, like those recommended in Chapters Two and Three, can enhance the power of any fertility treatment, boost your energy and, best of all, give you a feeling of control.

Chapter Six
· · · · · · · · · · · ·
Your Healthy PCOS Pregnancy

The great majority of women with PCOS can, and do, get pregnant. And when they do it can bring a whole load of emotions to the surface, from excitement to disbelief, panic to joy. Then, as you get used to the idea that you're going to be parents, you start wanting to read up about being healthy through your pregnancy – after all, you've heard of those extra risks of miscarriage and getting diabetes because of your PCOS. You worry that if you put on weight you'll never be able to get it off again because of the PCOS weight trap. And is the PCOS-friendly diet you've been following to keep your hormones in balance the best diet to carry on with now you're having a baby?

But hang on a minute – a lot of pregnancy books don't mention PCOS, so how do you know which bits of information are relevant to you or not? We hope this chapter brings you the PCOS-focused information you need to add to the general pregnancy wellbeing information already out there in all the books and websites. The basic ideas are the same – healthy eating, gentle exercise, and looking after yourself – but there are some extra steps you can take with PCOS to ensure you and your baby's health are the best they can be.

I'M PREGNANT! NOW WHAT?

First of all, you and your partner should congratulate yourselves and rejoice. Getting pregnant is a wonderful achievement and one to be proud of and excited about – especially if you have been following the PCOS fertility-boosting action plan. This has taken time and discipline and both you and your tiny baby-to-be are reaping the health-boosting benefits already.

IS THE PREGNANCY AT GREATER RISK?

If you've had trouble getting pregnant because of PCOS you may now feel anxious about staying pregnant. Your body didn't work as it was supposed to when you were trying to conceive, and more than an echo of the insecurity, the guilt and the worry can remain.

It might be logical to assume that PCOS is cured or goes away when you get pregnant, but there are still no straight answers to either of these questions. 'Although some women with PCOS find that their post-pregnancy cycles get more regular, there isn't any evidence that pregnancy cures PCOS,' says Adam Balen. 'What we do know, though, is that research does seem to indicate that a PCOS pregnancy is at greater risk.' While it may feel scary to read about these facts, knowing the risks means that you can deal with them in an active and positive way. So here's what we currently know.

It has been generally claimed that women with PCOS are more likely to miscarry than those with no PCOS.[222,223] There is an ongoing debate about this issue, and whether it is simply the fact that many women with PCOS are more likely to be overweight or obese, and thus these risks of increased miscarriage that are associated with the condition, or whether there is something more serious in terms of egg quality or hormonal imbalance that make a pregnancy less likely to succeed.

Outside of the risks associated with being overweight, Professor Stephen Franks says, 'Although it was thought that women with PCOS are more likely to have a miscarriage than those who do not have PCOS, recent evidence from large population studies suggest that women with PCOS are no more likely to miscarry than those without. That is supported by the results of the treatment programmes at St Mary's Hospital, London, for women with PCOS who require stimulation of ovulation. In short, there is no clear evidence for increased risk of miscarriage.'

However, other experts disagree, as a higher risk of miscarriage for women with PCOS has been attributed to higher luteinizing hormone concentrations in PCOS that could damage egg quality, and also to the weight management problems many women with PCOS have, as weight excess is associated with an increased risk of miscarriage.[224,225] In addition, there is also some evidence to suggest a higher rate of miscarriage for women who have become pregnant with assisted fertility treatments, like IVF.[226]

'Certainly, it appears,' says Dr Thatcher, 'that the risk of miscarriage is increased in mothers with PCOS, as are the risks of gestational diabetes, pregnancy-induced hypertension, unusually small or large babies and C-sections.' Some of these risks are linked to prepregnancy weight and others to insulin resistance, while the smaller growth may be specific to hormonal alterations in the PCOS ovary itself.

This all sounds alarming but it is important to point out that early miscarriage is far more common than most of us realize – regardless of whether or not you have PCOS. One study in 1996 looked at 200 women who were trying to get pregnant and found a 31 percent rate of early pregnancy loss.[227] But once you get past week 12–14, other research suggests that the pregnancy loss rate plummets to 1 percent and continues to fall still further as your pregnancy develops.

Check with your doctor

The latest research has thrown up some new questions you should talk through with your healthcare practitioner in the early stages of pregnancy.

- *Antidepressants.* Women using antidepressants are at a **68%** increase in risk of miscarriage, according to a recent study in the *Canadian Medical Association Journal.* Researchers from the University of Montreal analysed data from 5124 women who have suffered a miscarriage in the first 20 weeks of pregnancy. 284 (5.5%) of those who had miscarried had taken antidepressants during their pregnancy.

  SSRIs, especially Paroxetine and Venlafoxine, were associated with a higher risk of miscarriage. The author of the study says they can't make any definitive conclusion as to whether antidepressants increase the risk of miscarriage, but they warn there is a small risk. If you are taking them and trying for a baby, talk to your GP or specialist.
- *Being underweight.* Women who have a low body mass index before they become pregnant are 72% more likely to suffer a miscarriage in the first three months of pregnancy, but can reduce their risk significantly by taking supplements and eating fresh fruit and vegetables, according to study findings published online in *BJOG: An International Journal of Obstetrics and Gynaecology.*
- *High doses of caffeine.* High doses of daily caffeine during pregnancy – whether from coffee, tea, caffeinated soda or hot chocolate – cause an increased risk of miscarriage, according a new study by the Kaiser Permanente Division of Research. The study controlled, for the first time, pregnancy-related

symptoms of nausea, vomiting and caffeine aversion that tended to interfere with the determination of caffeine's true effect on miscarriage risk. 'If you definitely need caffeine to get you going, try keeping it to one cup or less a day. Avoiding it may be even better. Consider switching to decaffeinated coffee and other decaffeinated beverages during your pregnancy,' said Tracy Flanagan, MD, Director of Women's Health, Kaiser Permanente Northern California. 'Learn to perk up instead with natural energy boosts like a brisk walk, yoga stretches and snacking on dried fruits and nuts.'

The first three to four weeks are vulnerable for every woman but, if you've got PCOS, there's the added worry of your pregnancy being at even greater risk. So what can you do to ensure that you stay pregnant and your baby-to-be is in the best health?

In the positive pregnancy advice section below, we've outlined what you can and should expect from your healthcare provider if you have PCOS. We've also outlined things you can do to help with your pregnancy, some of which are just plain common sense and good for all women, but some of which are specific to women with PCOS.

YOUR POSITIVE PREGNANCY

What to Expect From Your Health Service If You Have PCOS

Every pregnancy carries with it risk, whether you have PCOS or not, but do you need to see a specialist in prenatal medicine if you have PCOS? The jury is out but most gynaecologists think probably not.[228] The important thing is that your doctor and you are aware that PCOS may increases your risk of certain pregnancy-related conditions and that your pregnancy is closely monitored. 'Although there can be medical complications that are more common to a PCOS pregnancy, and referral to a specialist may be needed, what is most important is that your health service provides education, answers to your questions, a process to allow early identification of potential problems associated with PCOS, and care for you and your partner as individuals,' says Dr Thatcher. 'There are increased risks with a PCOS pregnancy and appropriate monitoring should be provided,' says Adam Balen.

Pregnancy Tests

If you are past your due date it makes sense to do a pregnancy test before calling your doctor, as this is probably one of the first questions he or she will ask you.

Home pregnancy tests turn positive about the time of the first missed period or 14 days after ovulation. All pregnancy tests detect levels of human chorionic gonadotrophin (hCG) in your urine, resulting in a colour change of a specifically designed dye indicator. It is produced when the fertilized embryo implants in your womb lining and it is only present during pregnancy. Some women with PCOS say that the early hormonal changes of pregnancy often translate into fatigue, tender breasts and frequent urination.

Further Testing in the Early Weeks

After the pregnancy test, which is usually also confirmed by a blood test, your doctor may ask you to come back in one to two weeks to test your hCG levels again. Around two weeks after ovulation the hCG level should be 15–200 IU/litre. After this the level should double every 48 hours or so for the next two weeks – a multiple pregnancy would have a faster increase. Slower hCG rises or falling levels aren't a good sign and could suggest a possible pregnancy loss.

Your progesterone levels may also be measured at the same time as hCG and can help detect potential problems with the pregnancy, as progesterone is needed to sustain the pregnancy. If progesterone levels aren't reassuring (under 20 pg/ml), supplemental progesterone may be recommended until about nine weeks, when the placenta is able to make all necessary progesterone by itself and the ovaries aren't needed anymore.

How Pregnant Am I?

The typical pregnancy lasts 280 days, or 40 weeks from the last menstrual period – although, if your baby is born anytime between 37 and 42 weeks, this is entirely normal. Pregnancy is divided into three trimesters of around three months each. The first trimester is a time of rapid change and adjustment to the pregnancy. The downside is fatigue and possible morning sickness. The second trimester is usually the most enjoyable part of the pregnancy when complications are uncommon and a woman feels that pregnant glow. The third trimester can be very tiring and as delivery day draws closer most women have had quite enough of being pregnant.

Should I Have an Ultrasound Scan?

Ultrasound scans at around five or six weeks are usually routine to date a pregnancy, but perhaps the best reason for women with PCOS to have a scan is for the sense of relief it can bring.[229] If there is a problem, it's probably best to find out as soon as possible to see if anything can be done.

What Should I Do if I Start Bleeding?

Call your doctor immediately. Try not to panic. Rest. There will be bleeding in about one in three pregnancies and about half of these pregnancies will be lost, but bleeding does not always indicate that there's a problem. During implantation a small amount of bleeding or spotting may occur and it may occur again at the process of placental implantation. Generally, the greater the amount of bleeding and cramping the greater the chance of pregnancy loss.

TACKLING YOUR FEARS

So what are the real risks if you are a pregnant woman with PCOS and what can you do to ease them? Let's look at each risk factor in turn and see how you can help yourself, as well as what to expect from your doctor.

Gestational Diabetes

There haven't been any large scale studies but PCOS could increase the risk of gestational diabetes mellitus (GDM.) Gestational diabetes is defined as any degree of glucose intolerance during pregnancy. It is logical that women with PCOS, weight problems and/or insulin resistance are at increased risk of GDM and several small studies have suggested that around 45 percent of women with GDM have PCOS.[230]

GDM is one of the most common types of pregnancy complication and carries with it the risk of hypertension and caesarean section. You should be routinely screened for GDM by your health service provider between week 24 and week 28 of your pregnancy. But, since women with PCOS and insulin resistance are known to be at higher risk, you should ensure that you are screened as early as possible. It might also be a good idea to discuss routine testing throughout your pregnancy and after delivery. Contrary to popular belief, GDM doesn't always disappear when baby is born. It is thought that women with GDM have a 50 percent chance of developing type 2 diabetes within twenty years of childbirth.[231]

The usual way to screen for GDM is to perform a glucose tolerance test. You will be given a blood test after fasting from the night before, and then be asked to drink some glucose-rich liquid. A second blood test is taken after an hour to diagnose GDM. If the diagnosis is positive, diet restrictions will be recommended and you will be regularly monitored.

How is GDM Treated?

Though diabetic mothers and their babies were once at great risk, this is no longer the case, thanks to increased awareness of how to treat the condition. When blood sugar is closely controlled through diet and, if needed, medication, women with diabetes can and do have normal pregnancies and healthy babies.

If you have GDM you will probably see your doctor more often than other expectant mothers. You will be given more instructions and it's crucial that you follow them. Making a diabetic pregnancy a success will take a great deal of effort on your part, but the reward − a healthy baby − will make it worthwhile and there may even be an upside to all this diligent self-care during pregnancy. One study, FIND, showed that diabetic women took such good care of themselves during their pregnancy that they and their babies had even fewer problems than their non-diabetic counterparts.[232]

Close vigilance is required if you have GDM as high glucose levels can have a harmful effect on the growing fetus. Your doctor will give you strict dietary and exercise guidelines to control your glucose levels. There will be more frequent appointments with your doctor to check your glucose levels and at around 18 weeks an ultrasound will be given to screen for fetal health. Sadly, GDM carries with it a higher risk of miscarriage, especially in the third trimester, and self-testing of fetal movement is crucial. Your pregnancy will also not be allowed to progress much past 40 weeks.

There is no doubt that pregnancies with GDM are riskier but they can also be successful. Planning is everything. Hypertension, prematurity, unexplained fetal death and C-section are common complications, but these can all be avoided if attention is paid to diet and lifestyle recommendations, and regular tests and checks are performed.[j]

GDM Guidelines

The key to successfully managing a diabetic pregnancy is to maintain normal blood sugar levels. Below are components of a typical diabetic pregnancy programme designed to do just that. The programme laid out for you by your doctor may differ slightly, because it is tailor-made for you, and is the one you should follow – but the guidelines below give you an idea of what to expect if you are diagnosed with GDM. Whether you entered your pregnancy already with diabetes or developed GDM along the way, all the following considerations will be important in working towards a safe pregnancy and healthy baby.

A Good Diet

A diet geared to your personal requirements should be carefully planned with your doctor. It will probably be high in complex, low GI carbohydrates, particularly wholegrains, vegetables and beans (about half your daily diet should be from carbohydrates), moderate in protein (20–25 percent of calorie intake) and low in cholesterol and fat (30 percent of calorie intake but no more than 10 percent from saturated fat). Plenty of dietary fibre will be important (40–70 g daily are recommended since some studies show that fibre can reduce insulin requirements in diabetic pregnancies). All this advice is actually pretty similar to the advice on healthy eating that a woman with PCOS should follow anyway, so if you've been following the advice in the seven-step plan, you're well on the way to eating a healthy diet for your diabetic pregnancy.

As with all pregnant women you'll probably need around 300 extra calories a day, and an extra serving of protein (30 g), as well as regular healthy snacks made up of a protein and a complex carbohydrate component (such as celery sticks and hummous), to keep your blood sugar stable. You may need to watch the sugar content of fruit, as well, depending on how your body handles it.

Skipping meals or snacks can dangerously lower blood sugar levels so be sure to eat regularly, even if morning sickness makes you feel you don't want to. If you feel really sick, stick to bland simple foods, such as dry toast and crackers, and try to eat even when you don't feel like it – an empty stomach will just make the sickness worse. Getting sufficient calories is vital to your baby's wellbeing and never, ever try to diet during pregnancy. Weight gain should progress according to the guidelines set by your doctor, usually 25–30 pounds during the nine months. (For more on weight management in pregnancy see page 182)

Moderate Exercise
A moderate exercise program will give you more energy and aid in regulating your blood sugar, but it must be planned in conjunction with your diet plan by your doctor. Moderate exercise such as brisk walking, swimming and light biking might be suggested. Precautions you might be asked to observe when exercising include taking a snack before your workout, not allowing your heart rate to exceed 70 percent of the maximum safe heart rate for exercise for diabetic pregnancies, and never exercising in a warm environment.

Safe Exercise Heart Rate for Diabetic Pregnancies

To find 70 percent of your maximum safe heart rate for your age group, subtract your age from 220 then multiply your result by 0.70. For example, if you are 30, you would figure it this way:

220 minus 30 equals 190. Then 70 multiplied by 190 equals 130.

This means that 133 beats per minute would be your safe limit of exercise intensity and the level you should not exceed.

Rest and Relaxation

You might need regular rest and relaxation, especially in the third trimester. If you are working, your doctor might recommend maternity leave earlier than you may have planned, especially if your job involves standing, sitting or lifting.

Constant Monitoring

If blood sugar levels can't be controlled by diet and exercise your doctor might recommend that you take insulin medication. Try not to be alarmed if your doctor orders lots of tests for you, especially in the last three months, or even suggests hospitalization in the final weeks. This doesn't mean something is wrong; it just means that he or she wants to make sure everything stays right. Don't panic either if your baby is placed in a neonatal intensive care unit for testing immediately after delivery. This can be routine procedure for babies born to mothers with GDM.

Because babies born to mothers with GDM tend to be too large for full-term vaginal delivery and because the placenta often begins to deteriorate earlier, there is a possibility of delivery before full term at 38 or 39 weeks. This certainly isn't always the case though, and many women with GDM carry to full term safely.

Hypertension

Pregnant women with PCOS who are insulin resistant are also at an increased risk of hypertension or high blood pressure.[233] Hypertension is defined as a systolic pressure (top number) above 140 mm over a diastolic (bottom number) pressure over 90 mm.

Pregnancy-induced hypertension (PIH), also known as toxaemia, is the most common medical complication and happens in around 8 percent of pregnancies. It is responsible for 14 percent of all maternal deaths. PIH results in constriction of the vessels of the placenta, diminishing blood flow that can restrict fetal growth.

The placenta forms the interface between mother and baby and is the site where the complications of pregnancy that are associated with PCOS, such as hypertension and diabetes, can occur. It regulates the nutrient supply from the mother to the baby by accessing each of their needs and supplies. It plays a crucial role in pregnancy and any damage to the placenta will damage the baby.

Signs of PIH

Signs and symptoms of PIH include swelling of the hands and face, with sudden weight gain from water retention; high blood pressure – 140/90 or more in a woman who has never had high blood pressure – and protein in the urine. The condition needs to be treated immediately before it progresses to the more severe stage called pre-eclampsia, which is characterized by a further increase in blood pressure, blurred vision and headaches. Fortunately, in women who are receiving regular medical care the disease is invariably caught early and treated successfully, avoiding the rare bad outcome of it developing into full-blown eclampsia, which is characterized by convulsions and sometimes coma. Eclampsia can lead to permanent damage of the nervous system, blood vessels and kidney in the mother, and growth retardation in the baby.

Occasionally PIH doesn't appear until labour and delivery. It may be a reaction to stress or it may be true eclampsia. Therefore, women who have had elevations of blood pressure in their pregnancy are watched very carefully with frequent checks, and this is why, if you have PCOS and are therefore at a higher risk, it's worth talking this through with your doctor and making sure you're getting the right monitoring.

Treatments for PIH
If you do have high blood pressure, your treatment will vary according to how severe the PIH is, the condition of both you and baby and the length of the pregnancy. With mild disease you would usually be hospitalized for complete bed rest (lying on the left side is best as it takes pressure off the major vessels and allows maximum blood flow to the uterus) and close observation. In some very mild cases, you could bed rest at home once blood pressure has normalized. If you are allowed home you'll be monitored by a visiting nurse and will need to make frequent visits to the doctor. It's crucial you watch out for the danger signs – severe headache, visual disturbances, or upper or mid-abdominal pain – that can warn you that the condition is getting worse. Reducing salt intake can also help, as can preventing excessive weight gain in pregnancy. You might be given medication. Beta-blockers and ACE inhibitors have been linked to fetal death and the only safe drug for PIH is Aldomet. The only definitive treatment, though, is delivery, and in most cases hypertension disappears once baby is delivered.

Whether you're in hospital or at home, the baby's condition will be assessed regularly and, if at any point your condition worsens, or the baby is in distress and delivery is an option, then vaginal induction of labor is the usual next step. If you have PIH you won't be allowed to go past your due date since post term the environment in the uterus begins to deteriorate more rapidly than usual. Generally, the prognosis for a pregnant woman with mild PIH is good when medical care is appropriate, and pregnancy outcome is virtually the same as for a woman with normal blood pressure.

Natural Therapies for PIH

- A study by Professor Christopher Silagy and Dr Andrew Neil reported in the *Journal of Hypertension* in 1997 showed that garlic powder tablets have been proven to lower raised blood pressure.
- Hyperventilation (fast, shallow breathing), can push your blood pressure up, so learn deep breathing exercises and try to breathe from your abdomen.
- Colour therapy uses blue or indigo to lower blood pressure so wear these colours or put up a soothing picture in your living room.
- Yoga, tai chi and the Alexander technique if practised regularly could also help to lower blood pressure. Look out for special pregnancy classes at your local leisure centre.

None of the above should be used in place of a doctor's prescription if your doctor has advised antihypertensive drugs.

Obesity

As we have seen throughout the book, weight management problems and PCOS are closely connected and it seems that obese women with PCOS are at higher risk of complications of pregnancy when compared to obese women without PCOS. Many overweight women get pregnant and have healthy babies but obesity does increase the risks to mother and her baby.[234,235] The risks of obesity for pregnancy include hypertension, diabetes, caesarian section, birth defects, blood clots, anaemia, infection, more neonatal intensive care admissions and increased risk of postnatal death in the first week.

If you have PCOS, pregnancy isn't the one time in your life when you can eat what you like and not worry about your weight. Although dieting is not an option, you do still need to keep a close eye on your weight gain. Staying within the recommended weight gain for your height and prepregnancy weight is important for your baby's health and wellbeing. It's important for you too. Gaining too much weight now will increase your risk of GDM and PIH and make it harder for you to lose weight after your baby is born, setting you up for long-term weight management problems that can only make symptoms of PCOS worse. (See page 182 for our pregnancy weight management tips.)

Big Babies, Small Babies

The average birth weight of babies born to PCOS mothers doesn't seem to differ that much from those of the general population. Infants born before 37 weeks are said to be premature and they do not have the same risks as babies born small for their gestational age or growth restricted as a result of decreased blood supply to the placenta. There can be many causes of growth restriction but of most importance to PCOS patients are vascular problems arising from hypertension and diabetes.

Groundbreaking research by Professor David Barker at Southampton University, shows that what your baby weighs at birth can have a big impact on their health. There is a confirmed relationship between low birth weight and development of insulin resistance, hypertension, asthma and type 2 diabetes. Other findings suggest that low birth weight in a girl baby predisposes a woman to PCOS.[236,237] This is interesting as it would suggest that the development of PCOS has not so much to do with genetics, but more to do with prenatal stress, either from growth restriction, prematurity or from exposure to corticosteroids which are used to treat individuals at risk of preterm delivery.

Babies large for their gestational age are probably more common for women with PCOS. The major risks for large babies (macrosomia) are related to diabetes and obesity. Gestational diabetes is uniformly associated with bigger babies and, since PCOS and diabetes are related, it is reasonable to assume that PCOS patients not only have a greater risk of GDM but also of bigger babies.[238,239] Is it possible that being large for gestational age alters fetal metabolism to such an extent that it predisposes them to later development of PCOS? Could a glucose-rich environment in the womb cause insulin resistance and/or PCOS? No study has yet been done but it's an interesting connection.

Miscarriage

> 'I've had two miscarriages and I am worried about being pregnant again. My doctor tells me that it's nature's way but this doesn't help. I'm scared. I've got PCOS and my cycles are irregular and I'm overweight. Could PCOS be a factor in my pregnancy loss? What can I do to stop miscarrying again?' SUE, 36

The chance of a miscarriage for all pregnancies in all age groups is between 8 and 15 percent and that rate increases to about 15 to 25 percent in women aged over 35 and for those who have irregular menstrual cycles. Over 90 percent of miscarriages happen in the first 12 weeks but as the pregnancy progresses the rate of miscarriage decreases. About 15 percent of couples trying to conceive will have three or more losses, but even after recurrent pregnancy loss, the chance of pregnancy is still around 70 percent.

Early losses in the first 8 weeks are most often due to genetic and hormonal causes and poor egg quality. Between 8 and 14 weeks they might be due to uterine abnormalities. Loss in the second trimester might be due to disorders of the placenta and sometimes due to chronic disease. Losses in the third trimester are often maternal in origin and could be related to diseases of pregnancy such as diabetes and hypertension.

So, is miscarriage more likely if you have PCOS? We can't say yes for sure, as there is still a big debate about whether it is simply the fact that women with PCOS are more likely to be overweight or obese, and that these risks – which are relevant to any woman – are therefore increased. There are indications that women with recurrent pregnancy loss more often have polycystic ovaries on ultrasound. One of the most comprehensive studies, by a group led by Lesley Regan, reported on 2,199 women attending a recurrent pregnancy loss clinic in London. It found that 40 percent of the women had PCOS.

Is It My Fault?

It's important to know that, except in very rare cases, such as violent trauma or drug abuse, nothing you did caused the pregnancy loss. All patients with impending loss are placed on bed rest which leads many people to assume that activity increases the risk of miscarriage, but it doesn't. All that bed rest can do is ease anxiety and avoid the guilt associated with activity. Stress may have an adverse effect on pregnancy outcome and we'll discuss that in more detail below. Sex should be avoided as it can cause uterine contractions, but generally, once a pregnancy is established very little can be done to alter its course. 'Losing a baby is traumatic but don't let guilt compound your misery,' says pregnancy expert Heidi Murkoff, author of the pregnancy bible *What To Expect When You're Expecting*. 'A miscarriage is not your fault.'

Will I Conceive After Miscarriage?

The chances of you conceiving successfully again after miscarriage are good, at around 60 to 70 percent, even after three or four miscarriages. The risk of a second loss is only slightly higher after a first loss, and a high percentage of women who miscarry during fertility treatment will go on to have a healthy baby. Pregnancy often has a positive effect on reproductive health and some women with PCOS find that second time round they get pregnant easily. You shouldn't think that once fertility is impaired it always will be. 'Because of the hormonal shifts involved, a "pregnancy loss",' says PCOS expert Dr Thatcher, 'can sometimes have a positive effect on PCOS, making the next pregnancy both easier to achieve and more likely to be successful.'

'It's clear that providing treatment is continued, the chances of a successful pregnancy are much better than even,' says internationally respected infertility expert Professor Robert Winston. 'Remember that a miscarriage is sure evidence that your tubes are open, that you do ovulate and that the sperm is fertile.'

When Can I Try Again?

Your doctor will advise you on this. Generally, the advice is to wait three months to give women time to come to terms with the loss and for their menstrual cycle to re-establish itself. But the latest research suggests there may be no need to wait.

A team at the University of Aberdeen, Scotland, which studied 30,000 women, found that conceiving within six months offered the best chance for a healthy pregnancy. The findings, published in the *British*

Medical Journal in 2010, counter international guidelines that women should wait at least six months before trying again.

The researchers looked at data between 1981 and 2000 relating to women who had a miscarriage in their first pregnancy before going on to becoming pregnant again. Women who conceived within six months were less likely to have another miscarriage, termination or ectopic pregnancy, the figures showed. Also, conceiving within six months was associated with reduced risk of Caesarean birth, a premature delivery or a low birthweight baby compared with those women who had conceived between six months and a year.

But study leader Dr Sohinee Bhattacharya said that for older women, who are more at risk of miscarriage, a delay may actually hamper their chances of a successful pregnancy. 'Women wanting to become pregnant soon after a miscarriage should not be discouraged. If you're already over 35, I would definitely advise to try again within six months as age is more of a risk than the interval between pregnancies,' she said to the BBC. 'The only reason women may need to delay is if they have had a complication such as infection,' she advised.

PCOS AND BREASTFEEDING

There is currently a lot of debate surrounding the issue of PCOS and breastfeeding, as there are some experts, and women with PCOS who feel it can be made more difficult, for reasons as yet unidentified. One 2008 study from the Department of Laboratory Medicine, Children's and Women's Health, Norwegian University of Science and Technology, Trondheim, Norway, suggested women with PCOS appear to have a reduced breastfeeding rate in the early postpartum period.

Lisa Marasco, MA, IBCLC, is a lactation consultant in Santa Maria, California, and co-author of *Making More Milk*, who has studied the impact of PCOS on breastfeeding after suspecting a connection when two patients within a week show up with low milk supply and similar symptoms. She says, 'I looked at their history and found out they both had fertility issues and a diagnosis of PCOS,' she says. Building on her interest in low milk supply, Marasco decided to investigate the PCOS connection more thoroughly, making it the subject of her master's thesis. She studied a group of women with diagnosed lactation failure, and she found that PCOS was indeed a risk factor. Half of the women with lactation failure suffered from obesity, and 67 percent suffered from infertility – both of which are side effects of PCOS. Some women in her study group had never been diagnosed with PCOS but displayed symptoms and turned out to actually have the disorder. Marasco emphasizes, however, that PCOS affects all women differently. In a casual survey she conducted in an Internet PCOS support group, a quarter to a third of the respondents had supply troubles, and only a third of those had severe problems. 'A whole lot of them do fine,' she says. In fact, in a casual Internet survey she carried out, Marasco found that a percentage of the respondents actually suffered from oversupply.

There is no research yet that offers concrete proof of any link between PCOS and breastfeeding issues, just theories that a condition which interferes with hormonal health may be supposed to potentially have some effect. It is also noted that insulin plays a role in milk production, as women with uncontrolled type-2 diabetes mellitus often do not make enough milk, and therefore questions are being asked in many online discussion groups, about whether insulin resistance in PCOS might have an effect. For now, however, this is all supposition.

Professor Adam Balen says there is no evidence to support the idea that women with PCOS are more likely to struggle with breastfeeding. 'Currently there is only theory, without enough real scientific foundation,' he says, 'so we cannot draw any conclusions.'

What Can I Do?

'All mothers should be aware of their community breastfeeding resources, and they should not hesitate to contact a qualified counsellor if they are having problems,' says Lesa Childers, International Board Certified Lactation Consultant (IBCLC) and PCOS Support Chapter Development Coordinator, who is currently researching the link between PCOS and breastfeeding traumas. 'I would strongly encourage women with PCOS to line up a professional lactation consultant in advance, and to arrange for a consultation at the first sign of possible problems. Early intervention can be very important in some cases.'

Your doctor or local breastfeeding support group may be able to offer advice if breastfeeding isn't going as planned – just don't be surprised if the latter seems uninformed about PCOS. Once again, making contact with other women with PCOS and breastfeeding problems via support groups or online may be a source of advice and support.

Sometimes trying too hard can inhibit milk production, so it's important to back off and relax once in a while, and if that means giving baby a bottle then so be it. The breastfeeding 'police' are so adamant that breast is best it can leave mums who can't breastfeed or don't feel comfortable with it feeling inadequate, but every new mother needs to find what works best for her and her baby. 'When breastfeeding works it is indeed a glorious experience with many benefits to mother and child,' says Peggy Robin, author of *Bottlefeeding Without Guilt*, 'but if it doesn't work for whatever reason there are many positive aspects of life to a bottlefeeding parent and child, which in the current climate of "breast is best" tend to be forgotten or downplayed.'

WHEN CAN I STOP FEELING ANXIOUS?

You can't and you won't. There won't be a time in your pregnancy when you will feel completely anxiety free, whether you have PCOS or not. That's the nature of motherhood. There is always another hurdle to face, whether it is getting pregnant, hearing the fetal heartbeat for the first time, seeing your baby move on the ultrasound screen, feeling it move in your womb; delivering a healthy baby at birth; feeding; the first day at home, walking, talking; potty training; the first day at school; exams; first boy or girl friend; exams again or the eighteenth birthday. You will always worry about your kids!

SEVEN STEPS TO BOOST YOUR HEALTH AND WELLBEING DURING PREGNANCY

What happens to you – what you eat, what you breathe, the good and bad experiences you have – can affect your unborn baby right from the date of fertilization, when it's too small to see with the naked eye, for the rest of his or her life. Don't let this panic you, as nobody can do the right thing 100 percent of the time, but do let it encourage you to do your best for your baby and yourself.

When you get pregnant, probably the best thing you can do is be diligent about seeing your doctor, report anything that seems unusual, eat well, pace yourself but still get good exercise, and do all the things that should be done by any pregnant woman who is determined to take good care of herself and her unborn child. Use the seven steps to a positive pregnancy below, as a reference to keep you on track.

Step One: Carry on Eating Healthily

As always with PCOS, get your diet and nutrition on track. Good nutrition is the key to everything in your body. Dieting during pregnancy is definitely not on. Just keep eating healthily.

Why It's Important

Your baby's health is programmed in the womb. Researchers are learning that the developing baby-to-be is much more sensitive to the mother's nutritional status than previously thought. Experts from St Thomas' Hospital in London believe that the health of the mother during pregnancy affects our health just as much as the life we lead as adults. Mothers who eat for two and consume a diet too high in saturated fat could be putting their unborn babies at risk of heart disease, diabetes and high blood pressure later in life. Poor intake of one or more essential nutrients during critical periods in an organ's growth can alter the structure, size and function of that organ. There could be serious health consequences later in life.

Babies born to mothers who are not eating properly and giving their baby-to-be all the nutrients he or she needs are often born larger or smaller than they should be. The nutritional deficiencies associated with larger or smaller babies can have a big impact on their chances of survival after birth and their future health.[240]

Some experts believe that large birthweight babies (over 8 lb 8 oz) are at greater risk of developing breast cancer in later life. Babies born weighing less than 6 lb are at greater risk of being premature or stillborn, or having poor development, lowered intelligence and neurological problems, and learning difficulties. 'Inadequate nutrition is associated with an increased risk of growth problems, or what is known as fetal growth restriction,' says Bruce Shephard MD, Clinical Associate Professor of Obstetrics and Gynecology at the University of South Florida College of Medicine.

There may also be a link between high sugar diets during pregnancy and spina bifida.[241] The latest research also shows sugary colas are linked to gestational diabetes (drinking more than five servings of sugar-sweetened cola a week prior to pregnancy appears to significantly elevate the risk of developing diabetes during pregnancy, found research published in the journal *Diabetes Care* in 2009), and type-2 diabetes outside of pregnancy. If, for example, you aren't eating well when your baby's pancreas is forming and its size, structure and function is affected, it could be at greater risk of developing diabetes as an adult.

It's clear that good nutrition is vital for a healthy pregnancy and a healthy baby. But according to a 2004 survey of 1,000 women commissioned by the makers of Sanatogen ProNatal, a multivitamin supplement specially tailored for the needs of women during pregnancy, even women without PCOS don't know what to do about nutrition during pregnancy. So what if you have PCOS as well?

What Dietary Changes Should I Make?

If you've been following a healthy diet, like that in our PCOS fertility-boosting action plan while you were trying to conceive, good for you. Keep it going now you're pregnant. It might also be a good idea to ask your doctor for pregnancy diet information and advice, and mention your increased risk of gestational diabetes at the first meeting. Even if you haven't got gestational diabetes, you may want to eat a diet for people with diabetes as a preventative measure. The pregnancy diet for diabetes is complete and offers good nutrition.

You may be surprised to learn that, if you're already eating a healthy diet before you became pregnant, you probably won't need to change it that much to cover the extra nutritional demands of pregnancy. This is because your body adapts during pregnancy and becomes very efficient at absorbing and retaining nutrients. Pregnancy is a time of extremes. You have never been so excited. You have never been so tired. You have never been so hungry. But surely it's okay to eat a lot. After all, aren't you eating for two?

Yes, but don't go overboard. Remember your baby-to-be is very,

very tiny, not the size of the Incredible Hulk! Your unborn child only needs an additional 300 calories a day, and that's only in the last two trimesters.

Step Two: Manage Your Weight

Excess weight has been linked with symptoms of polycystic ovaries. Obesity, as well as too much weight gain in pregnancy, have also been linked to health issues for mother and baby during pregnancy – from pre-term and low birth weight babies, to an increased risk of having an infant with a neural tube or heart defects, as well as more than doubling the risk of obesity in children; and for the mother, an increased risk of gestational diabetes, raised blood pressure, pre-eclampsia and the need for a Caesarean section, as well as an increased risk of being obese 16 years after the birth. So weight management during pregnancy is vital for your health and the health of your baby-to-be.

In the past, when we didn't know quite so much about our bodies, gaining considerable weight when having a baby may have seemed inevitable. But today, with a basic understanding of how to work with your changing body during and after pregnancy, it is possible to gain a healthy amount of weight to ensure the health of your baby but also to retain your figure after the birth so symptoms of PCOS are less likely to return. Post-baby fat is not impossible to shift if you follow some basic pregnancy weight management guidelines during and after pregnancy.

Pregnancy Weight Management Tips

Try to stay within the recommended range of weight gain for pregnancy for your height and build. Research has shown that, if you gain the recommended amount of weight during pregnancy, you are less likely to have a permanent struggle with extra weight later.

So how much weight do you need to gain to satisfy your baby's needs as well as your own health needs? And what if you entered your pregnancy already overweight? The Institute of Medicine in Washington DC recommends a weight gain of 25 to 35 lb during pregnancy. It also recommends different weight gain guidelines based on your weight and height before conception.

Pregnancy Weight Gain Guidelines

- If you are underweight for your height (BMI less than 19.8), or if you are a teenager, the recommended total weight gain would be between 28 and 40 lb.

- If you are normal weight, your recommended total weight gain would be between 25 to 35 lb.

- If you are overweight (BMI over 26), your recommended weight gain would be between 20 (15 if you were obese) and 25 lb. However, your doctor may recommend that you gain less weight than this, depending on your individual circumstances: the latest expert thinking is questioning whether currently recommended weight gain is sometimes necessary.[242]

- If you are expecting more than one baby your weight gain guidelines need to be discussed with your doctor, but are usually in the range of 35 to 45 lb.

It's important for all pregnant women to pay attention to these guidelines but it's particularly important if you have PCOS – being overweight during pregnancy increases the risk of miscarriage and makes post-birth weight loss harder, and so can trigger or make symptoms worse. So ignore all those well-meaning friends who encourage you to indulge by telling you that you're eating for two, and that this is the one time in your life you don't have to worry about your weight.

But don't restrict your intake either – even if you entered your pregnancy overweight. Dieting during pregnancy is completely not on. If you gain under 20 lb, your baby is more likely to be premature and at risk of growth problems. Your baby needs a constant supply of nutrients every day and can't get all he or she needs from your fat stores. Your baby needs you to be well nourished. If you are not he or she will suffer. If you gain the recommended amount of weight for your height and build, you are most likely to produce the healthiest weight babies. Babies born at optimum birthweight (6–8 lb) have the lowest risk of developmental disorders.

Around 20 lb of the weight you gain is for your baby's development. You don't have much control over that. Maternal fat over and above what your baby needs accounts for 5 to 10 lb of your overall weight gain. These additional pounds prepare and strengthen your body for the demands of the growing baby. The excess fat also helps nourish you and your baby in the final months of your pregnancy and during birth and breastfeeding. You do have control over the additional amount of weight you gain here, but it is believed that an extra 5 to 10 lb of maternal fat increases your chances of delivering a healthy birth-weight baby.

Why You Need to Gain Weight

There is a use for every pound you gain when you get pregnant. The weight you put on is not all for your baby and neither is it all fat. If you were to gain 27 lb your weight gain would break down like this:

Baby	7.5 lb
Placenta	1.5 lb

Fat and protein stores	7.5 lb
Blood volume and body fluid	6 lb
Amniotic fluid	1.5 lb
Breast tissue	1 lb
Expanded uterus	2 lb

How You Should Gain Weight

How you gain weight during pregnancy is almost as important as how much weight you gain:

The First Three Months

During the first three months you should ideally be gaining between 1 and 4 lb. You don't need to eat more than you normally do at this time, you just need to make sure your diet is healthy and nutritious (see page 206). Your doctor or midwife will also give you a diet sheet with recommended amounts of protein, carbohydrate and fat and other pregnancy food guidelines.

From Three to Six Months

This is the optimum time for you to gain weight, as your baby needs an increased food intake and you should be eating an additional 300 calories each day. These calories should come from healthy, nutritious food choices like a wholemeal salad sandwich and a glass of milk. Weight gain at this time should be at a steady rate of 1–2 lb a week.

From Six to Eight Months

From six to eight months you should continue to gain about 1 lb a week, with weight loss slowing in the ninth month. The second trimester is the time of rapid weight gain. The third trimester is the time for slowing down, conserving your energy and preparing for the baby.

Although these guidelines sound very specific, they're just to show you that a small increase in weight has a point to it and will help you and your baby-to-be. Excess weight isn't an inevitable consequence of pregnancy for women with PCOS. Every woman is unique and it's impossible to stick rigorously to these guidelines; such an approach could increase your stress levels and be detrimental to both you and your baby.

There will be times when you gain more weight than others, and morning sickness, fluid retention and food cravings can all cause fluctuations in your weight gain. Keeping an idea in your mind, however, of the kind of weight gain to aim for can alert you to potential problems (weight gain that is too slow or too fast can be an early warning sign of problems with the pregnancy), and help you avoid overeating and gaining too much weight which isn't good for you or for your baby.

Step Three: Get Rid of Unhealthy Habits

Avoid cigarette smoking, alcohol consumption and caffeine. You don't need anything that could compromise your pregnancy or make symptoms of PCOS worse.

Smoking

Smoking suppresses your appetite, robs your baby-to-be of vital nutrients and can interfere with your ability to eat enough food. You also increase the risk of miscarriage, preterm delivery, and a low birth-weight baby. You would have to be blind, deaf and dumb not to know the harmful effects smoking can have on a developing fetus. Pregnancy is a time for new beginnings and what better time for you to quit this dangerous and harmful habit, for both your health and the health of your baby-to-be?

If you smoke and want to quit, talk to your doctor. Starting an exercise programme will help with weight management. Be sure to take a multivitamin too. There are many ways to give up smoking, but perhaps the most effective is to simply stop. The nicotine will pass out of your system within a few days. When you crave a cigarette after that, you are not craving nicotine but the habits you associated with nicotine. What you have to do now is try to find other habits to replace the smoking habit. With a baby coming into your life, this shouldn't be too hard. There are a million and one things for you to think about and do – you haven't got time for cigarettes anymore!

Alcohol

Any alcohol that you drink during pregnancy is passed through your placenta into the baby's bloodstream. No one is really quite sure what the safe limit is, so it's best to avoid alcohol altogether and make your own fresh cocktails, milkshakes, and sparkling mineral water drinks instead. Even beers, lagers and wines that claim to be alcohol free, or low in alcohol, are not necessarily free from harmful additives and chemicals that can have unknown effects on your baby-to-be's health.

Babies born to heavy drinkers can have what is known as fetal alcohol syndrome when growth and intelligence is affected. Even a moderate amount may harm your baby-to-be. All pregnant women are advised not to drink when pregnant. One recent study concluded that alcohol intake during pregnancy can increase the risk of pre-term birth.[243] If you enjoy alcohol, talk to your doctor about the risks.

Caffeine

The latest research concerning caffeine intake during pregnancy is fuelling the debate about whether it makes any real difference or not. One recent study suggests it does not encourage pre-term birth or low birth weight babies[244], whereas two others suggest even small amounts could restrict the growth of a foetus, and affect the development of the foetal heart.[245,246] The experts are still debating this issue.

We do know that caffeine withdrawal can affect newborns and cause feeding difficulties, colic and irritability. Because of the uncertainty concerning how harmful caffeine is, it is probably wise to keep your consumption down – say no more than two cups of coffee a day.

Drugs

All drugs are dangerous for your baby-to-be. Within 30 minutes of ingestion or injection they are in your baby-to-be's blood too. Just don't take them. If you do have an addiction or dependence problem talk to your doctor immediately.

Medications

All medications, whether over-the-counter or from your doctor, are potentially harmful during pregnancy. Always discuss with your doctor any medication, painkillers or dietary supplements you are taking, to ensure they are safe to use in pregnancy.

Unsafe Food

Foods to avoid during your pregnancy include 'junk food', highly seasoned food, caffeine, fried foods and rare or undercooked meat, poultry and shellfish. Grilling can produce harmful substances in meat, so avoid it. Especially avoid raw eggs, raw meat and unpasteurized foods like soft goat's cheese and mould-ripened cheeses, such as brie and blue cheese, which may have been infected by harmful organisms. Cottage cheese and hard cheeses, however, are fine. The Food Standards Agency also recently advised pregnant women to avoid entirely mercury-contaminated fish, such as tuna, swordfish, shark and marlin.

But Don't Be a Saint!

Just because you're pregnant doesn't mean you have to become a food saint. If you enjoy chocolate, ice cream and other foods that are high in fat and sugar, go ahead and eat them. If about 90 percent of your diet is healthy and nutritious you can afford to spoil yourself once in a while. A balanced diet contains a wide variety of foods – even chocolate contains antioxidants that are now thought to be good for you. Just don't go overboard – you can enjoy a little of everything in moderation. One bar of chocolate, not five. One scoop of ice cream, not the whole carton.

Step Four: Exercise Regularly and Gently

We've seen how important regular exercise is if you have PCOS and as part of your fertility-boosting action plan. It is also significant when you get pregnant.[247] For a start, regular exercise while you're carrying your baby will improve its heart health. A 2008 pilot study conducted by Linda E. May, exercise physiologist and anatomist at Kansas City University of Medicine and Biosciences found that pregnant women who exercised at least 30 minutes three times a week had fetuses with lower heart rates – a sign of heart health – during the final weeks of development. A 2011 study from the same team, presented at the Experimental Biology 2011 annual meeting in Washington, DC, has revealed that the fetuses' improved cardiovascular heart control is maintained one month after pregnancy, which indicates that mothers' efforts to stay active have lasting effects.[248]

You may worry that you'll feel too tired. Physical changes will make it hard for you to move, bend and even breathe. You're going to gain weight anyway. So why bother keeping fit when you're pregnant?

Why Exercise In Pregnancy?

- It keeps your muscles, bones and heart strong
- It stimulates your metabolism so that you burn calories faster — helping you maintain a healthy weight throughout the nine months
- It improves your sense of physical and emotional wellbeing, by helping to relieve backache, prevent morning sickness, varicose veins and constipation, as well as lifting your spirits and easing stress
- It makes it easier for you to get fit and slim again afterwards — vital if you've got PCOS — and to be an active carer for your child
- There is evidence that exercise during pregnancy can reduce the risk of diabetes — women with PCOS are at an increased risk of this

If you took a nine-month break from any type of exercise you'd be much less fit afterwards. It would take quite a while to get your form back. Although you won't be able to train vigorously when you are pregnant, you can still maintain your fitness levels — or boost them if you're not very fit at the moment — so that returning to normal activity afterwards is a smoother transition, which will be better for your health, better for your child and for your relationship, social life and work. You'll also be maintaining the healthy habit of exercise as a PCOS-fighting tool to help keep any symptoms under control once you've given birth. If you didn't exercise before pregnancy, now is not a good time to start a strenuous programme, but on the other hand pregnancy is no reason to put off being active.

Is Exercise Safe During Pregnancy?
During the dark old days when having a baby was considered an illness, you weren't supposed to exercise. Now we know better and

the American College of Obstetricians and Gynecologists encourages expectant mothers to keep active – it does you and your baby good.

The only way you put your baby-to-be in danger is if the activity is exhausting, strenuous and violent, such as running a marathon or climbing a mountain – not if it is moderate. Moderate activity in a healthy, well-nourished expectant mother can actually prevent health problems like excessive weight gain, poor posture and back pain and a poor body image, something many of us with PCOS have enough trouble with as it is.

As long as you have no obstetric or medical complications, including those below, you can continue to exercise and derive benefits. If you have achieved cardiovascular fitness prior to pregnancy, you should be able to safely maintain that level of fitness throughout pregnancy and the post-partum period.

Always seek advice before doing any exercise if you suffer, or have suffered in the past, from:

- pregnancy-induced hypertension

- preterm rupture of the amniotic sac and leaking of amniotic fluid

- preterm labour during a prior or the current pregnancy, or both

- incompetent cervix cerclage (the procedure by which the cervix is stitched closed after conception)

- persistent second or third trimester bleeding

- intrauterine growth retardation (inadequate development of the fetus or placenta)

- a history of miscarriage in the first trimester.

There is no research to prove that fit women have easier pregnancies and deliveries but many doctors feel that fitness helps women cope better with the demands of pregnancy. In the words of Dr Arlene Jacobs, obstetrician and gynecologist at the Plano Medical Center in Plano, Texas, 'It is safe to exercise when you are pregnant. For all pregnant women, especially women with PCOS, I recommend regular exercise. I'd only have reservations if a woman has never exercised before. She must start very gradually and slowly.'

However, do consult your doctor before you begin any exercise programme in pregnancy. It is also wise to discuss continuing any exercising you were doing before you got pregnant. He or she will be able to discuss with you any medical circumstances that might have an impact on your working out. Certain conditions, such as those listed above, may require you to modify your exercise programme or to avoid exercise altogether.

Fit To Be a Mum
You may feel that simply being pregnant is enough of a workout for your body. You would rather rest than go for a walk or a jog. That's fine. You don't have to exercise when you are pregnant. It's just that regular exercise will help manage your weight and strengthen your body for the demands of pregnancy, childbirth and post-partum recovery.

Try to think of these nine months as a training period. You are training to have a baby. You are training to be a fit mum. You don't want to be listless, stiff and out of condition when your baby-to-be arrives. One of the greatest gifts you can give your baby is to be fit and alert enough to welcome him or her with energy into the world.

Step Five: Reduce Stress
We've seen how damaging stress can be for you if you have PCOS and

how it can negatively impact on your fertility. Not surprisingly, it isn't good when you're pregnant either. There is a wealth of international research from America, Ireland, Spain, France, Australia and Britain suggesting that babies are aware of their mother's emotions in the womb: that a relatively calm pregnancy tends to produce calmer babies, and that a stressful life during pregnancy can affect a baby's neurological circuitry for good.[249] This can have many different potential effects ranging from impaired ability to deal with stress, to hormonal disorders like PCOS.

Stress isn't good news if you are undergoing fertility treatment either. A study published in March 2004 suggests that psychological and relationship problems cause many couples to stop having fertility treatment. Researchers in Sweden surveyed 974 couples who were having IVF. Writing in the journal *Fertility and Sterility*, they said 26 percent of these dropped out for psychological reasons while 15 percent were having marital problems.

Cut down on stress in all areas of your life. Make room for your pregnancy. Don't power on regardless. Take time consciously to relax for a minimum of 20 minutes every day. And as you do, visualize your baby safe and secure and happy in your womb.

Communicate With Your Baby

International research suggests that spoken and unspoken (happy thoughts) communication between mother and unborn baby can begin as early as the first few days of conception. Why not take a few moments each day to do a simple visualization exercise like the one below?

Close your eyes, breathe deeply and in your mind's eye see your baby nestling safely in your womb lining and staying there, growing, safe and secure. Send messages of love, happiness and welcome to him or her, telling them they are safe, loved and wanted. And if you, or your partner, talk aloud or play calming, uplifting music (Mozart is often recommended) to your unborn child, prenatal research from Ireland suggests that your baby can hear as early as 17 weeks, even though the actual ears don't form until week 33.

Mother Yourself

Take some time for yourself also. Your pregnancy can be an amazing opportunity to learn the importance of self-nurturing and plant the roots of self-love so deep that, when you become a mother, you will be able to replenish yourself and give authentically to your child without losing yourself.

'Every woman not only richly deserves self-care,' says Jennifer Louden, author of the bestselling 'Comfort' books, 'but she must have it if she is to survive and thrive as a mother. Pregnancy offers us the excuse to be gentle on ourselves. That excuse can become a habit. That habit can slowly become a lovingly held belief: "I am worth self-care, not just when I am carrying a child, but every day".'

Although you probably feel as if all your time and attention should go on your growing baby, some time and attention must be given to you too. Many mothers say that they wished they had taken advantage of their pregnancy more. For some reason it didn't dawn on them that this might be the last time in quite a while when they could take it easy. So during your pregnancy, repeat to yourself over and over again: Enjoy this time. Slow down and relax. It may never come again. Of course you want to keep your baby's welfare firmly in mind, yet it is vital for you also to emphasize your needs.

Mothering yourself and reducing stress means taking time for yourself and doing what makes you feel good. Sometimes in the flurry of responsibilities we forget how to make this possible. Use the suggestions below as a starting point to weave relaxation and enjoyment into your life.

Relaxation Tips For Pregnancy

LET GO OF THE 'SHOULDS'   Every time you catch yourself saying or thinking I should do that, try changing the should into a could to see if that helps reduce feelings of stress.

MAKE RELAXATION A HABIT   Try taking a mini-relaxation every time you need to use the restroom. Making relaxation a habit prepares you for labour, when knowing how to relax can help you in a big way. When you sit down, consciously relax your shoulders and jaw. Close your eyes and breathe deeply (hopefully the restroom will be clean), and say silently to yourself a calming word, for example peace, or love or chocolate. Then exhale through your mouth and repeat several times.

THINK POSITIVE THOUGHTS   When you feel conflicted, stressed and unable to relax indulge in some positive self-talk. Many inner voices are critical or negative but pregnancy provides a unique inner voice, which can calm you and remind you of what is important. Find a few moments when you can be alone. Close your eyes and concentrate on breathing deeply from your belly. Feel the breath going down into your belly. After a minute or two, let any thoughts that occur to you to come to mind. It might be: Why can't I relax? or it could simply be: Good morning. Now relax and let the energy of your pregnancy answer your question. Don't strain. Just tune in. You'll almost certainly get a 'be good to yourself' answer. Try it and see. An example is on page 196.

AND WHAT ABOUT DADS-TO-BE? Stress related to pregnancy uniquely affects the health of expectant fathers, which in turn, influences the health of expectant mothers and their infants, says a 2011 University of Missouri study, which recommends that health services should incorporate counseling and assessments for men and women to reduce stressors and promote positive pregnancy outcomes, says ManSoo Yu, assistant professor in MU's Public Health Program. So get your partner involved in managing his stress, too.[250]

Positive Self-Talk

I feel stressed.   Breathe. Take it easy. Feel the new life inside you.

I feel so tired.   Focus on the new life inside you. Take some time out.

I'm afraid.   Don't pressure yourself to feel happy all the time. Find what makes you feel good and stop worrying about what you should and should not do.

Finally, if you really can't relax, allow yourself to be good to your soon-to-be child. Motivate yourself by reminding yourself: my baby needs me to sit down or relax or be good to myself. After you get used to this, try again to transfer this caring behaviour to yourself. Visualize how connected you are with your baby. Feel in your heart that caring for and loving your baby cannot be separated from caring for and loving yourself. When you take your prenatal vitamins, whisper some positive thoughts to yourself, such as: I feel honored and special to be a mother.

REMIND YOURSELF OF YOUR ACHIEVEMENTS   Every time you feel your baby kick, think of all the times in your life when you have felt proud of yourself.

Small achievements count just as much as big ones, and it doesn't have to be to do with your pregnancy.

PRAISE YOUR BODY   When you walk or use the stairs, remind yourself that your body is keeping two people alive. Praise your body and congratulate yourself on keeping active.

DO SOMETHING SPECIAL FOR YOURSELF   After each prenatal appointment do something special for yourself. Perhaps you would like a pedicure or perhaps you'd like to spend a few hours browsing in your local bookstore. It doesn't matter what it is as long as it makes you feel good.

KEEP A PREGNANCY JOURNAL   Buy a special notepad and pen and keep a journal of pregnancy. Record your hopes and fears, your thoughts and dreams. Pregnancy is a time ripe with insight so write down what you want to when you want to. It will help calm you and help you celebrate and make sense of your experience.

STRENGTHEN THE SUPPORT AROUND YOU   Pregnancy offers a unique opportunity to create or strengthen your support team so that it is in place post partum for when you really need it. When you are pregnant you'll find that it's easy to connect with other women, make new friends and meet new people. New mums, loving friends, an understanding family and of course an understanding doctor and midwife are essential for your medical and physical and emotional health, both during and after pregnancy. And allow your support team to nurture and support you. People who care about you are generally really happy to listen, hug, reassure or lend a helping hand so you can put your feet up and relax.

Step Six: Check Out Complementary Therapies

Perhaps you have used complementary therapies to help treat symptoms of PCOS or to boost your chances of getting pregnant. You might like to think about carrying on with some during your pregnancy. Pregnancy brings with it a host of uncomfortable physical symptoms, from haemorrhoids to heartburn. And just when you need them the most, conventional drugs are off limits. Even 'take two aspirins' is no longer a safe option. Yet help is available, say fans of complementary medicine. Natural therapies offer some of the safest, and often only, ways to get relief.

Morning Sickness and Nausea

Laura, 37, felt so nauseous during her second pregnancy that she couldn't leave home for fear of fainting. 'The doctor could only prescribe bed rest, but that wasn't an option with a 14-month-old to look after,' she says. A friend persuaded her to visit a naturopath. 'Within days of following the naturopath's advice to take regular vitamin and mineral supplements, drink lots of dried ginger root tea and press acupressure points at the base of my wrist, I felt better.'

Terrible feelings of sickness and nausea are thought to affect over 80 percent of pregnant women in some way. Doctors can't offer any approved pharmaceutical treatment but research shows that natural therapies may offer relief. A study reported in the *Archives of Gynecology and Obstetrics* talked about a significant reduction in nausea and vomiting in women who took vitamin and mineral supplements; a study of 30 women suffering from nausea who took part in trials recorded in the *European Journal of Obstetrics and Gynecology and Reproductive Biology* found relief from taking 250 mg of ginger in capsule form four times a day; and the conclusion drawn in the *Journal of the Royal Society of Medicine*, by at least seven randomized trials of acupressure and acupuncture for pregnancy sickness, is that it can work.

'Citrus oils such as grapefruit, lime or lemon, or peppermint, can ease nausea during pregnancy, and labour,' says Denise Tiran a practising midwife, university lecturer, Educational Director of Expectancy (www. expectancy.co.uk), and author of professional textbooks including *Clinical Aromatherapy in Pregnancy and Childbirth*. 'Put one or two drops on a tissue, and inhale as needed.'

Complementary Therapies and PCOS Pregnancy

'Most of the pregnant women I treat have been to their doctors first,' says homeopath, nurse and antenatal teacher Anna Foxell, who treats pregnant women in Windsor and Harley Street, London. 'They have been down the conventional road, and it hasn't helped them. Pregnancy is the ideal time to discover the benefits of alternative therapies, not only because drugs are off limits, but also because, when a woman is pregnant, she tends to be more open to new things. I've found that the cure rate during pregnancy is much higher. You have to drop your defences in order to unconditionally love a child.'

But are complementary therapies safe during pregnancy if you've got PCOS? On the whole, natural therapies can't harm a pregnant woman or her baby-to-be, but problems arise when alternative practitioners unknowingly give pregnant women with PCOS the wrong herb, dose or advice. So do your research. Natural therapies can be brilliantly useful during pregnancy if you take them with caution and under supervision from your healthcare practitioner/pharmacist, and always read the label.

More and more experts are taking this view including Dr Tanvir Jamil, co-author of *The Alternative Pregnancy Handbook* and a practising GP with specialist knowledge of complementary medicine, and obstetrician Yehudi Gordan, who founded the St John and St Elizabeth's Hospital's Birth Unit in 1981 (where midwives and obstetrician recommend, in addition to conventional care, a network of complementary therapists, including osteopaths, Ayurvedic practitioners, homeopaths, aromatherapists, nutritionists, acupuncturists and self-hypnosis therapists). 'We view these therapies as extremely powerful aids for pregnancy, labour and postnatal health,' says Gordan.

Treatments to Avoid

Certain herbs, essential oils, and nutritional supplements can be as potentially harmful as drugs during pregnancy – tansy, sage and large doses of vitamin A, to name but a few – and normally safe therapies can be extremely dangerous. For instance, naturopathic treatments that include fasting, going on a restricted diet, or even drinking lots of water to relieve heartburn and flush out toxins. The fetus needs a steady supply of nutrients, and more than two litres of water a day can overburden the kidneys. Hydrotherapy, which involves alternating hot and cold baths, can promote healing, but raising body temperature above 100.4°F is not recommended during pregnancy. Some traditional Ayurvedic medicines may contain mercury and lead – dangerous during pregnancy. Yoga, massage and acupuncture can relieve stress, but only in the hands of practitioners skilled in the treatment of pregnant women.

Alternative therapies should not be used carelessly at any time, especially when a woman is pregnant. 'Natural' does not always mean 'safe'. Conventional pharmaceuticals and treatments must undergo rigorous clinical trials to demonstrate safety before being licensed as medicine, but the majority of herbal remedies and alternative therapies are exempt. How then can a pregnant woman know the therapy she chooses is safe? She should check with her doctor and make sure she works with a qualified practitioner of alternative medicine. 'All registered therapists must subscribe to the Code of Conduct agreed with the Royal

Midwife Association,' says Paula Marie from the British Complementary Medicine Association. 'Therapists can't treat a pregnant woman without agreement from her midwife or doctor first. There should be no treatment at all in the first three months, during labour and 10 days after and no physical therapies, like massage, from the seventh month.'

Complementary therapies may help you stay well and have a smoother, calmer pregnancy and labour but always check first with your doctor and your complementary practitioner for safety of use during pregnancy. The following treatments have been recommended and used during pregnancy by women with PCOS:

Complementary Therapies Recommended For Pcos Pregnancy
ACUPUNCTURE AND ACUPRESSURE   Acupuncture can be used to treat numerous problems in pregnancy, for example aches and pains, morning sickness and headaches. The main advantage is that it is safe to use during pregnancy and breastfeeding and brings relief to pain that is unresponsive to conventional therapy, thus enabling a decreased use of painkilling tablets. It gives a feeling of relaxation after therapy and works well with conventional therapy.

ALEXANDER TECHNIQUE   The Alexander technique, with its emphasis on correct posture, is excellent for almost all aspects of pregnancy, especially back pain, pelvic floor strengthening, tiredness, stress, anxiety, low mood and headaches. The main advantage of the Alexander technique is that there are plenty of local courses available where you can learn the technique and eventually practise it for yourself without the presence of a teacher. The exercises should be done twice daily for 10 to 15 minutes.

KINESIOLOGY   Kinesiology is a system of manipulation and massage that can be particularly useful for backache, neck pain, stiffness, tiredness and depression. It's excellent for helping aches and pains during pregnancy and after your baby is born.

AROMATHERAPY   Aromatherapy is now so popular in pregnancy and labour that many midwives often include its use in their advice for antenatal classes. Some midwives also practise aromatherapy themselves and will use it to help you to make childbirth a positive experience. The advantage of aromatherapy is that the basics are easily self-taught from books or local courses. Do bear in mind that there are certain essential oils you cannot use at all during pregnancy, such as sage, clove, cinnamon, fennel and tarragon, and some you shouldn't use in the first trimester, such as rosemary and peppermint. Always make sure you check for contraindications.

'For many years I have seen essential oils have profoundly helpful effects during pregnancy and birth, from lavender offering relief for low back pain in late pregnancy, to jasmine helping to relieve the pain of labour, and clary sage being used by qualified practitioners to help bring on contractions,' says Denise Tiran, a practising midwife, and author of professional textbooks including *Clinical Aromatherapy in Pregnancy and Childbirth*. 'But I realise there are challenges for women who want to use them, not least buying reputable products, getting up-to-date expert advice, and finding a properly qualified practitioner.' For anyone wanting to use aromatherapy, Denise recommends using books that are less than two years old, and asking any practitioner for a certificate of insurance and details of their experience because aromatherapy is not legally regulated (for pregnancy and birth, check they are insured for work specific to pregnancy and contact the Federation of Ante-natal Educators for more advice: www.fedant.org). 'Buy essential oils in small dark glass bottles as they are damaged by light and air,' she says, 'and choose a reputable company.' Another buyer's tip is that some essential oils, such as jasmine and rose, are usually more expensive than lavender or tea tree because it takes much more of the raw ingredient to produce a drop of oil. If all the oils in a range cost around the same price (£5 or £6), check the labels as some may already be diluted with a carrier oil.

'Perhaps most importantly,' says Denise, 'I would urge anyone using aromatherapy oils in pregnancy to be cautious, and to do so ideally with expert guidance, because they are powerful substances that have a profound effect.'

BACH FLOWER REMEDIES   The following remedies are suitable for symptoms in pregnancy:

- Rescue Remedy for emotional and physical stress

- olive for tiredness

- crab apple for morning sickness

- aspen for anxiety

- mimulus or walnut or rock rose for fear

- mustard for depression.

The advantages of Bach Flower Remedies are that they are simple to use at home and are widely available from health food stores.

HERBAL MEDICINE   Herbal medicine can help many of the uncomfortable symptoms of pregnancy. Try:

- ginger and chamomile for morning sickness

- lime flower for stress

- peppermint for indigestion

- psyllium seeds for constipation

- yarrow tea or cranberry juice for cystitis.

The advantages of herbal medicine are that it is safe, if prescribed by a professional herbalist. Do make sure, though, that if you have been taking any herbal supplements prior to getting pregnant you discontinue them until you have checked with your doctor and a qualified herbalist.

HOMEOPATHY   Homeopathy is very safe and can help a lot of pregnancy-related symptoms. The advantage of homeopathy is that there are very few side effects. To get the maximum benefit from any remedies, do make sure you see a qualified homeopath experienced in treating pregnant woman before self-prescribing.

HYPNOTHERAPY   Many women find hypnotherapy helpful during pregnancy. It can ease stress, morning sickness, pain and low mood. It can also help increase your confidence and change unwanted bad habits, like swearing and smoking. The advantages of hypnotherapy are that it is easily taught and good practitioners are easy to find.

MASSAGE   Massage is one of the best therapies to use in pregnancy because it is safe, little equipment is required and expectant mums often experience positive feelings and a sense of calm during and after the massage. However, as with all physical therapies, it should not be used after the seventh month.

MEDITATION Meditation will help keep you healthy and happy if you practise for around 10 to 20 minutes every day. It's easy to learn and do and can be used for specific ailments such as nausea, stress, high blood pressure, fatigue and low mood.

NATUROPATHY The advantage of naturopathy is that it is safe during pregnancy. Common sense diet and lifestyle changes, like those given above, will be recommended to support the health of yourself and your child. If you have been taking any nutritional supplements or it is suggested that you do, check with your doctor to see if they are safe to take during pregnancy.

REFLEXOLOGY Reflexology can be particularly helpful for a whole host of pregnancy-related symptoms such as headaches, nausea, anxiety, constipation and aches and pains. It is gentle, calming and relaxing.

OTHER THERAPIES We've listed the therapies most suitable for women with PCOS above but there are many other complementary therapies that are now commonly used during pregnancy. These include yoga, t'ai chi, colour therapy, rolfing, shiatsu, osteopathy, chiropractic, Ayurveda and autogenic therapy. (For more information on all the above complementary therapies see our Resource Guide on page 275)

Step Seven: Listen To Your Body

As long as you don't go to extremes there is no evidence to suggest that work or exercise or travel have an adverse effect on pregnancy. Stress is a big danger but you can find ways to deal with that. Pregnancy is not an illness and, although you might find it harder to get around, you can do much that you normally did.

Don't Push Yourself

If you're worried that you might do something to endanger your baby, stop short and don't push. This could mean taking some time off work, dropping a commitment or changing your routine. Above all, listen to your body. It will tell you when you aren't taking care of yourself. If you're tired, rest; if you are hungry, eat; and if you feel stiff, have a stretch. If you're worried about anything talk to your doctor. If you think you could have a problem, get it evaluated. In the past, you may have been able to struggle on regardless when symptoms of PCOS flared up or you felt unwell but you simply can't do that anymore. Life isn't just about you anymore – it's about you and your future child.

In trying to have a successful pregnancy, it's easy to lose sight of the object of all this planning and attention. Becoming a mum is both exciting and daunting, but try to remember that from now on your child relies on you for love, security and the best that you can give.

AFTER THE BIRTH

Don't forget that taking good care of yourself by eating well, exercising regularly, managing your weight and watching your stress levels is just as important now as it was before and during pregnancy.

Keep on Eating Well

A healthy diet is extremely important after you've had your baby. 'The baby more or less "vacuum cleans" the mother in terms of nutrients, whilst in the womb and breastfeeding,' says nutrition expert Oscar Umahro Cadogan, who is a lecturer for the Danish Institute of Optimal Nutrition. Umahro urges all new mothers to make sure they continue to eat healthily once baby is born, not just because a breastfeeding baby's health and wellbeing depends on proper nutrition, but because the mother's health and wellbeing do too.

The fact is that many women get completely run down by pregnancy and breastfeeding. It's important that once baby is born, or when you have stopped breastfeeding, that you carry on eating healthily. If you've got PCOS, good nutrition and managing your weight is just as important now as it always has been. Be especially careful to eat healthily in the first six months post partum to take advantage of the weight loss window discussed on page 209. And after that, keep on eating healthily, (according to the healthy eating guidelines we gave in Chapter Two), to help manage your symptoms.

Keep Active Too

Exercise may be the last thing on your mind with a new baby to care for 24 hours a day, but it really is crucial for weight management and to boost your health and wellbeing. In the first few weeks, gentle walking is enough but, once you've had your six-week check up and the doctor is happy with your progress, there is no reason why you shouldn't gradually increase your exercise levels so that you are exercising for 30 minutes or more four or five times a week.

Bye, Bye Baby Fat

The first six months after birth is your weight loss opportunity. Research into post-partum hormonal changes reveals exciting news for women with PCOS: at no other time in your life is your body so efficient at weight loss, and at no other time is there such an opportunity for you to override your 'set point' – the weight your body always seems to return to after you lose weight. You could even end up weighing less than before you got pregnant.[251,252]

Your Weight Loss Opportunity

In the first few post-partum months your body is primed for weight loss. This is because during this time your fat-burning, appetite-suppressing hormones are activated. Normally your internal chemistry favours weight gain, as every woman with PCOS who has tried to lose weight knows too well. But now for around six months things are very different. When you give birth oestrogen and progesterone levels plummet but your metabolism remains high. It takes an average of four to six months for your hormones to get back to their pre-pregnancy state, longer if you're breastfeeding, and these six months of hormonal adjustment give you that unique chance to lose weight and perhaps reset your set point.

So how do you take advantage of this weight loss window? Remember things are different now. Your body is primed for weight loss and searching for balance, so you don't need to diet or restrict your food intake drastically. All you need to do in those six months is to relax and eat a healthy, nutritious diet – like the one we outlined in our PCOS fertility-boosting plan.

Don't Crash Diet

Crash dieting is a mistake as this will simply confuse your metabolism. It could trigger a starvation response where you cling to fat, which sets you up for long-term weight management problems. You may feel uncomfortable with the extra weight you have gained during pregnancy and want to lose it all as quickly as you can, but dieting and vigorous exercise right now is the worst thing you can do. Just eat healthily, exercise gently, be patient for a few months and let your body do the rest.

Many women with PCOS who eat healthily during the post-partum period find that weight management is less of a problem post baby than it was before they got pregnant. And if your weight is under control you're less likely to get as many PCOS symptoms – could this be the reason why some people claim that having a baby cures PCOS? The six-month weight-loss window could be the reason why their symptoms don't return to the same extent after a baby.

How You Can Expect to Lose the Weight
Typically, after delivery you can expect to lose around 12 lb. This isn't the 20 or so pounds you may have hoped for but don't worry, in the weeks that follow you will continue to lose weight gradually if you just choose simple nutritious foods and get your body moving with gentle walking. This will encourage you to lose weight as naturally and as quickly as possible.

In the next six weeks you enter another round of weight loss and will usually lose an additional 9 to 12 lb. After that, any weight loss is baby fat (the weight that remains won't fall off automatically and it's up to you to gently work it off), but remember that for up to six months post partum your hormones are still working in your favour so, as long as you keep eating well and exercising gently, the weight will melt away.

A combination of dieting and exercise is a more effective way of losing weight after pregnancy than dieting alone, concluded a recent Cochrane Systematic Review of available research.[253] By studying data from six different trials that involved a total of 245 women, researchers found that women who did exercise did not lose significantly more than women who have a standard post-natal lifestyle. But women who combined exercise and dieting did lose more weight than those with normal care.

'As well as helping reduce body weight, exercise has the added advantage of improving the women's cardiovascular fitness and preserves muscle – dieting alone reduces muscle mass,' says Amanda Amorim, an epidemiologist working in Rio de Janeiro, Brazil.

Losing weight isn't always easy with a new baby to care for, but your health and wellbeing should be just as important now as your baby's. Perhaps you could ask a friend or relative to look after the baby for an hour or so, so you can shop for some healthy foods. Or perhaps you could take your baby for a walk every day to make sure you get some gentle exercise.

After six months – usually around the time periods and/or symptoms of PCOS return – your hormones settle down into their usual pattern and it won't be as easy to lose weight. Don't panic, though, if after six or seven months you still haven't lost all the weight, because you have an opportunity to rethink your approach to body image and weight loss. You have a new baby, a new body and a new life so forget the old rules. In your new life as a mother you don't diet anymore – dieting belongs to the past – you eat healthy, nutritious foods that are good for you. You keep active to encourage your body to be fit and healthy, and most important of all you keep a sense of perspective and enjoy the way you look.

Make Sure You Support and Take Time for Yourself

Looking after a new baby is stressful and lonely at times, and you'll need all the support you can from your partner, your friends and your family. It's especially important for you and your partner that you share the child care together, involving them in your life and feelings. Don't just divert all your emotions to the baby.

Finally, remember the advice about mothering yourself we gave earlier. Try to carve out some time for yourself every day. A new baby can be all consuming but you also need to find some time to mother yourself. This can be as simple as a relaxing bath at the end of the day, or doing something you enjoy, like reading a book, listening to music or spending time with friends when baby naps. Or perhaps you could ask a friend or family member you trust to look after your baby for a few hours so you can go out for a meal with your partner, get some exercise, go shopping, indulge in a massage or simply have some time for yourself. Yes, there may be 101 things on your housework and baby 'to do' list and it may seem indulgent to spend time on yourself, but always remember that the greatest gift you can give your baby is a healthy, happy and relaxed mum.

Good luck. Here's to your child of the future. May he or she be healthy and happy and bring you much joy.

Chapter Seven

• • • • • • • • • • • • •

Riding The PCOS Emotional Rollercoaster: Staying Sane and Happy Through Your Fertility Journey

'I remember the first time that I saw infertility and PCOS marked as my diagnosis ... certainly it did not apply to me. But as each failed cycle went by, I was forced to realize that yes, I had PCOS and I may be infertile. A strange condition to accept when I had always imagined myself with at least three kids, and yet the reality of being able to do that now seemed beyond me.' ANN, 29

Worrying about whether you should or indeed can have a child can bring up a whole range of emotions, from anxiety to despair and anger to depression, as well as delight, excitement and joy. If anxiety about your fertility is making you feel confused and vulnerable, or if you are undergoing fertility treatment and finding the whole experience traumatic and invasive, read on for positive ideas about how to cope with the emotional rollercoaster.

There are three main areas that bring their own peculiar set of emotional ups and downs when you have PCOS and you're tackling the issue of fertility.

AREA ONE: BIOLOGICAL CLOCK ANXIETY – SQUARED!

The phenomenon of biological clock anxiety is a fairly new trend as women put off having children for much longer than we did a generation ago. But with PCOS, the effect of wondering when is the right time to have a baby is intensified by the worries about how long it might take to get pregnant.

Previously medics had thought that a woman's fertility started to decline in her thirties, but findings from researchers at the University of Padua, Italy, and the National Institute of Environmental Health Sciences in North Carolina, US, suggest a woman may start to find it harder to conceive in her late twenties. And according to fertility experts at the University of Utrecht in Holland, women who delay babies for career reasons should be told how falling fertility levels could hamper their chances of having a child later in life.

So what happens if you get diagnosed with PCOS and suddenly you're faced with the prospect of fertility problems? The fear of being robbed of any choice in the motherhood issue can often prompt women with PCOS to make decisions much earlier than we would have liked.

If you've got PCOS, there is no escaping the fact that from the age of 35 at the latest you really do need to confront the issue of whether or not you want children. But what if you really don't know? There are tools and techniques recommended by experts to help women cope with biological clock anxiety. For instance, talking to women who have chosen not to mother or become mothers can be very helpful in offering insights into the consequences of that choice. Spending time with children to see what you are letting yourself in for can also be useful. But although helpful, none of these techniques can really help you answer the most important question: how much do I really want a child? If you are nearing readiness to make a decision here are the kind of questions you should be asking yourself:

Questions to Ask Yourself About Becoming a Mother

- Are you prepared for the possible discomforts of pregnancy and child birth?
- Are you willing to open up your relationship or marriage to a third party?
- Are you prepared to devote the first few months of your baby's life entirely to him or her?
- Are you prepared to feel lonely and isolated at times?
- If you plan to raise a baby alone, are you prepared to endure criticism and are you willing to accept that it will be harder for you to find a partner?
- Are you willing to embrace the chaos a child brings: the sleepless nights, the loss of free time, routine, control and personal space?
- Are you prepared for the overwhelming responsibility of a child?
- Have you thought about the bad as well as the good possibilities? What if your baby has a health defect, your partner leaves, and you lose your job?
- Are you prepared to love your child whatever its sex, temperament and personality, not just as a baby, but as a child, a teenager and a young adult?
- Are you prepared for the cost and extra expense a child can bring?
- If you are going to continue working are you prepared for the stresses of juggling home and career?

If you don't feel ready, or if your lifestyle isn't conducive to a baby, or if you are not at all sure you want to have a baby, it makes sense to wait, even though PCOS and declining fertility may be urging you to make your mind up. Talking to friends, your partner, and loved ones who you feel will understand you, or seeing a counsellor or therapist can be helpful. It's also well worth investigating the issue with other women in a PCOS support group or specific biological clock anxiety support groups, like those run by RESOLVE in the USA.

What About Waiting?

The idea of having children can often override whether or not you actually want to have children and will be a good mother. The purpose of therapy, counselling, support groups or talking things through with an understanding friend or family member is not for you to resolve all your emotional conflicts but to help you decide what you really want, so that PCOS or other people don't pressure you into a decision.

Giving yourself permission to wait does carry the risk that you may not be able to have a child in the future and, if this happens, regret and sadness are inevitable, but always remember there were reasons for the choices you made. If you're worrying about how much time you might have left, experts still believe that your easiest indicator of predicting your age at menopause is asking your mum when she started hers. And as we'll see in the next chapter there are other ways to bring children into your life, such as adopting, fostering or mentoring. There is so much emphasis on pregnancy and giving birth that it overshadows the fact that it is what happens to children after they are born that really matters.

Ambivalence About Motherhood

As you explore the issues, you may even find that children are not for you. Deciding not to have children involves coping with the inevitable fear of missing out later in life, although you can also think of all the energy, time, freedom, experiences and extra money you will have. Remember that mothers have their regrets and frustrations too. No life choice is perfect. There is no reason why a woman without children should feel alone. The number of women remaining childless by choice is increasing. According to the US census takers nearly 20 percent of women in the baby boomer generation are not having children. The US now has a child-free network with over 50 meeting places for child-free couples. The organization believes that child-free people should be respected for who they are and not be judged by whether or not they have children. A child-free life can be full, productive and happy, and should be carefully considered if you feel ambivalent about children. In the UK, the charity ISSUE has set up an organization for child-free people called More to Life, an exciting new development which aims to build a network of support across the UK for the growing number of child-free people. If you have chosen not to have children it might be worth contacting them for advice and support. (See our Resource Guide on page 275)

We are a lucky generation of women. We may not have it all but we have a lot. Those of us with PCOS can lead a full and interesting life with or without kids and, thanks to fertility drugs and treatments for PCOS, we have choice. But like it or not, PCOS brings the spotlight on to your fertility and, by so doing, it is instrumental in prompting you to make decisions about what your priorities and possibilities in life are. By focusing on what you want from life and how important motherhood is to you, you can emerge with a stronger sense of identity. Seen in this light the 'baby or not' issue becomes an exciting voyage of self-discovery where you set the course for the rest of your life.

Medical Breakthrough

A new test may soon be able to tell a woman the age at which she'll become infertile, i.e. go through the menopause. Dr Hamish

Wallace from Edinburgh's Royal Hosiptal for Sick Children led the research, which was reported in the *Journal of Human Reproduction* in June 2004 – with computer expert Thomas Kelsey from St Andrews University. Kelsey says the technology exists and could be made available to GP surgeries and fertility clinics in the next couple of years, and could be a first step in family planning. It can be used on young girls as well as older women and uses ultrasound to predict how many fertitle years a women has left. It can't, however, be used by women who are on the pill as hormone-based treatments suppress the ovaries. This could revolutionize family planning for all women and be extremely helpful for women with PCOS who are concerned about how fast their biological clock is ticking and how much they have left before it runs down.

AREA TWO: TRYING FOR A BABY

If you do decide to or are currently trying for a baby, having PCOS can add an extra dimension of worry and anxiety to the whole process, with the constant 'will it happen?' question going round your head. It can make sex and your relationship stressful; you can feel under pressure to do everything right with your diet, exercise and lifestyle because you know it will be of benefit; and if you're not careful, every little thing you feel you haven't done perfectly can make you feel a failure – whether it's not exercising one night because you're tired, or craving a junk food meal the next, to that ultimate feeling of frustration when your period arrives once again and you know you're still not pregnant.

For couples going through this process it can be good to know that other people are too. Joining a support group, meeting other couples experiencing similar challenges can be a huge relief.

'Hooking up with couples who were going through what we were going through really helped us feel less isolated. It also helped us see that there was a funny side to it. For example, when I'd phone my husband in the middle of a meeting with his bank manager because I was at my peak fertility and he had to make hasty excuses and rush off. Laughing about it broke the tension and helped us have better, less functional sex.'
BRYONY, 34

You can get information and support from organizations set up especially for couples having problems getting pregnant (see Resource Guide on page 275). Or you may prefer to get some support from a relationship counsellor or sex therapist. Having an objective third party can help you talk more openly. If that all sounds too daunting or too public, there are many useful books for couples with relationship or sex problems or for couples going through fertility treatment. You could simply schedule some time for you both to sit down and talk and read about your problems together.

The main thing is not to get so obsessed with the fertility aspect of your life that everything else suffers. Follow the 80/20 rule when it comes to eating well and exercise. Doing well 80 percent of the time is enough and gives you the room for treats and a night off. Think about the fact that it takes average couples without PCOS around a year to get pregnant and you can take the pressure off yourself in terms of how fast you expect pregnancy to happen. And most of all, reassure yourself that over 70 percent of women with PCOS do get pregnant naturally, so the odds are in your favour.

AREA THREE: THE HIGHS AND LOWS OF FERTILITY TREATMENT

If you decide that you do want kids and are considering or undertaking treatment for infertility, don't underestimate the emotional impact of your treatment. Finding out that you need medical help to have kids is a crisis and one that will probably take you by surprise.

> 'When we got married,' says LAURA, 34, 'we expected to start a family within a year. I knew a couple who were going for IVF but I never thought it would happen to us. It was a huge shock when I was diagnosed with PCOS. Equally shocking was the realization that once we began treatment our problems weren't solved. I thought that medical science had an answer for everything. I thought Clomid would do the trick. It didn't. Then I assumed IVF would make it happen. It didn't. I'm about to begin my third cycle of IVF next month and am beginning to realize that doctors still don't know that much about the seemingly simple task of getting pregnant.'
>
> 'We were so anxious and unhappy and moody and worried about money, that after three cycles we decided to take some time off and discuss if it was all worth the heartache. That really helped, because spending time together made us see that, however much we wanted a baby, we still wanted to be with each other more.' MARIA, 39

'Coping with fertility treatment can be like coping with bereavement. Couples go through as many emotions – shock, anger, denial – every single month,' says childcare expert and author of *Infertility: The Last Secret*, Anna McGrail. The constant failure as month after month goes by can strike deep at a woman's sense of self and there may be days when all the joy seems to go out of life. You may even wonder, like Mary, whether you should continue treatment: 'The struggle takes over your life. I often stop and wonder how life might have been if I was normal and could have babies easily. Some days I wonder why I am punishing myself over and over again when I may never conceive. I'm tired of living in a permanent sense of crisis.'

Acknowledge the Stress

Fertility treatment can take over your life, interfering with your relationships, your sex life and your work. The whole invasive process can be exhausting and expensive. Many women say that they find their world shrinks. Timing is crucial if the drugs and treatments are to stand a chance of success and all your attention needs to be focused on getting it right. According to Alice Domar, Director of the Mind/Body Center for the Women's Health Program at the Beth Israel Deaconess Hospital, Harvard Medical School, women trying unsuccessfully to get pregnant can have stress levels, in terms of anxiety and depression, equivalent to women with cancer, HIV and heart disease.

'Conception can become the main focus of your life, putting you on a roller coaster ride that ends with dashed hopes once a month when your period arrives. Tracking ovulation can take all the fun and spontaneity out of sex and marital disruption is common,' says Joan Borysenko.

Many women are prepared to risk everything if there is even a tiny chance of becoming a mother. There is always the hope that maybe next time the treatment will work.

'We tried for two years before seeing a doctor. When I was diagnosed with PCOS I freaked out. I've always wanted babies. What if I'd left it too late? We had test after test after test and five cycles of Clomid. Still no baby. Even more heartbreaking, on one cycle I did get pregnant but

miscarried at week ten. I really lost it then. It took a lot of courage to start another cycle, this time on Pergonal. Thank goodness I did because it was the cycle on which I finally conceived my son.' NICOLA, 35

'When we decided to start a family I knew that PCOS might cause problems so I went to see my doctor right away. I was 36 and my doctor warned me that there could be problems. After I don't know how many cycles of Clomid I was told that I needed to see a specialist, but because of my age the NHS couldn't treat me. Even if I had been younger I would still have had to wait years on the waiting list. Steven and I decided to take a risk and pay for private treatment. We were very lucky. I got pregnant with twins. I know lots of people who have several courses of IVF and don't get pregnant but it worked for us first time. Life's wonderful now.' LAURA, 37

The Waiting

Harder still is the constant waiting. Waiting for appointments, tests, referrals, more tests, results of tests, more tests, results of tests, a medical procedure, the results of the procedure, funding decisions, treatment options, ovulation, results, more tests …

Agree on a Limit

There is also the decision of how far you are prepared to go with your treatment. If you are an NHS patient in the UK, funding will, of course, determine the the limit. If you pay yourself, most clinics will recommend four treatments with IVF. If you want to keep trying and trying, much depends on how much your body and mind can endure, but it is important that you know when to stop trying – and that you remember you do have a choice. If you are in a relationship, communication with your partner is vital – both must agree what the limit is. If you are single, you need to have an idea in your mind of how far you are prepared to go.

Coping with the stress, anxiety, shock and uncertainty of fertility treatment is exhausting and stressful. It can damage your self-esteem and your relationships. What makes it harder is the fact that many couples are reluctant to talk about their problems, preferring to keep things to themselves, but isolation at a time in your life when you feel most vulnerable is an added burden.

'I just can't talk to anyone about the way I feel. We keep things very quiet. If things go wrong I don't think I could cope if people know. Trouble is I feel as if I'm living a lie. People say how lucky we are to have our freedom and to take all those holidays. How could I tell them what we really want is a child to share our "wonderful" life with?' LILY, **38**

STAYING SANE, HAPPY AND POSITIVE THROUGH THE FERTILITY JOURNEY

So, how do you manage the emotional rollercoaster of any one of these PCOS fertility situations? How do you ensure you don't feel isolated or guilty or totally controlled by unpredictable emotions? This four-step action plan can help you to weather the storm in a positive frame of mind.

Step One: Building Your Self-Esteem

Your sense of womanhood and femininity can get a bashing when you have PCOS and its symptoms, such as excess hair, male pattern baldness, weight gain that hides female curves and no periods. How do you deal with these and the assault you can feel on your femininity if you are finding it hard to get pregnant, or trying to get pregnant with the shadow of that hanging over you?

> *'I don't feel attractive any more. Getting in the mood for sex is really hard. All I see when I look in the mirror is this shapeless, plump woman with a light moustache and thinning hair. I can't understand what my husband sees in me. I don't have periods and because of that I don't feel like a proper woman. I've always wanted a large family. Now I'm not sure if I can get pregnant. I feel like a failure. My body isn't working properly. I don't feel feminine.'* SOPHIE, 34

When your body doesn't do what it is expected to do, or you don't look the way you think you should look and you feel your body has betrayed you, your self-esteem can take a huge knock.

'Your level of self-esteem,' says Boston psychotherapist and author of *Women and Self-Esteem*, Linda T Sanford, 'affects virtually everything you think, say and do. It affects how we see the world and our place in it. It affects how others treat us, the choices we make, our ability to give and receive love and our ability to take action to change things that need to be changed. If a woman has an insufficient amount of self-esteem, she will not be able to act in her own best interests.'

Low self-esteem can gradually destroy the quality of your life. You start to take less and less care of yourself. Your relationships, your sex life and your work suffer. You sell yourself short by deciding that you aren't good enough before you start anything, which means you don't put the effort in and end up fulfilling your idea that you aren't any good.

A healthy sense of self-esteem when you decide to go ahead with fertility treatment is important. Fertility treatment is a huge commitment to make and you need to feel good about yourself to maximize your chances of success – remember how damaging emotional stress can be to your fertility. Accepting that you have self-esteem issues and tackling them now can help you avoid a downward spiral. It's been said many times before, but thinking positively and putting more emphasis on the good things in your life is a great way to build your self-esteem. No one says this is easy but here are a few ideas to get you thinking along the right lines:

Think and Talk in a New Language
'You feel the way you think,' says clinical psychiatrist at Stanford University School of Medicine in the US, Dr David Burns. 'Negative feelings do not actually result from the bad things that happen to you but from the way you think about these events.' If you think and talk negatively or always put yourself down, you will sooner or later end up believing those thoughts. A powerful self-esteem booster is to make an effort to fill your thoughts and language with positive, liberating messages. For instance, avoid saying 'I can't' or 'I'm useless' and replace it with something like, 'I'll try my best' or 'I am getting better'.

Accentuate the Positive
Turn problems into challenges and fear into excitement. Avoid 'should' and 'ought' and replace with 'could'. When something goes wrong, remember to put it into perspective. It is one event and doesn't mean you will always get it wrong. Don't think 'I've failed' think 'I'm learning new things all the time and I'll know better next time.' Don't think 'I've got PCOS, I'm never going to lose weight and I may not be able to have babies.' Think 'PCOS is encouraging me to take better care of my health and appearance and focusing my attention on how I can maximize my chances of having a healthy baby when, and if, the time is right.'

Bring Fun and Laughter Into Your Life
You are bound to feel better if you do. It's all too easy to get stuck in a complaining rut and focus on the down and serious side of life. Make room for some playtime, whether it's watching your favourite comedy, seeing a friend who always lifts your spirits or reading your favourite book. And smile more. Smiling can help you stop feeling bad about yourself and encourage others to communicate with you.

Teach Other People How to Treat You
If people aren't valuing you, it's because you're letting them. Ask yourself why you're allowing this to happen and change the relationship by changing your behaviour. Act assertively and people who treat you like a doormat will either change their behaviour or leave your life. An assertive woman knows what she wants and respects her own wishes; she believes she can make things happen and does them; she isn't afraid to say no or take a chance; she accepts responsibility for her actions, expresses her true feeling and respects and values the feelings of others. Above all, though, she values herself.

Do Something
If you've been promising yourself that you'll learn a new language, start a new course, decorate your room, get a new wardrobe or style makeover, phone your parents, clean the house or take a holiday, make sure you stop procrastinating and do it. Get rid of guilt and get started. You'll feel so much better and this good feeling will encourage you to make even more positive changes in your life. Try doing something creative like painting a picture or writing a letter or baking a cake. It's amazing how quickly our interest in life can be recaptured when we encourage ourselves to be creative. And why not do something you have never done before? Encourage your natural curiosity – it may be a concert,

an activity, a trip or a class. When we do something for the first time, we always experience a charge of energy and learn new things about ourselves.

Write an Appreciation List

If you are feeling low, find things, no matter how small, to appreciate. You may have to search hard but it is worth the effort. The act of appreciation is the foundation stone of self-esteem.

Be Kind to Yourself

The next time you feel pleased with yourself because you've done something well, reward yourself with a treat, a trip, a meal or some leisure time. If you don't think you do anything well, then spend time focusing on your strengths. Write out a list of all the things you know you are good at, from dealing with people to making a chocolate cake or being on time. You'll be surprised at the lift it gives you when you concentrate on your positive strengths.

Stop Comparing Yourself to Other People

Remember you are unique. There never was and never will be another person on this planet like you. This makes you one of kind, special. Whenever you feel the urge to fit in, accept and make the most of your differences. They are what make you a unique and original person with your own place in the world.

Don't Put Off Life

Don't wait until you lose weight, have a partner, get pregnant, or get a promotion to love yourself. Start loving yourself today. Tell yourself over and over again that you are loveable for who you are, not for what you look like or what you do. At first it may seem weird and unbelievable, but do it often enough and it will start to become a habit. And when things become a habit they become part of who you are. Self-confidence is our birthright – just look at any newborn baby: it wants and expects love. Lack of self-confidence is something that has happened to you along the way and become a habit – perhaps because of negative messages that were given to you. Break that habit and replace it with the habit of self-confidence. After all, it is your birthright.

Become Your Own Best Friend
When you feel really low, try this wonderful technique to lift you out of your negativity. Imagine that you have stepped out of your body and are standing next to yourself. Become your own best friend. Now, what would you say to yourself that is comforting and helpful? How can you encourage this person to feel more confident about herself? What would you say to your best friend? Perhaps you would put your arm around her and tell her that she is doing really well and that you appreciate all the good things about her. Talk to yourself the way you would to your best friend.

Take a walk in the park...

...and you'll boost self esteem and happiness, say researchers who discovered that exercising in green surroundings for just 5 minutes a day had a miraculous effect on mental wellbeing.[254] Working in the garden, or walking a nature trail or other green space also counted.

Body Image
Working through the PCOS issues surrounding your body image is an important part of building your self-esteem and nourishing your sex

life. Body image and self-esteem are intimately linked. The danger lies in letting your negative attitudes towards your body colour your sense of yourself as a failure in all aspects of your life.

The great majority of women worry about the way they look. A 2003 nationwide survey of 45,000 women carried out by Women's Channel at AOL, found that only 4 percent of women were happy with their looks and around two-thirds feel uncomfortable with the way they look. Worrying about body shape was an everyday occurrence for 41 percent of women, with 26 percent saying it bothered them most when clothes shopping.

Most of us aren't entirely happy with our bodies, from ears that we think stick out to a stomach that sags. Other people may not think the same thing and see us far less critically and this is the difference between our bodies and our body image. 'Restoring and maintaining a positive body image when you have PCOS, especially when you are trying for a baby, can be extremely hard. And putting on weight, finding excess facial hair, losing hair from your head, dull skin, acne and worrying about fertility due to absent or irregular periods can all have a hugely damaging effect on your body image,' says Dr Helen Mason, Senior Researcher at St George's Hospital medical school, London.

There are two important steps you need to take if you want to feel less negative about your body. Learning to be happy with the body you have is one of them, and forgiving your body for not looking the way you think it ought to look is another. These are very difficult processes to try and work through but they are by no means impossible.

A positive body image makes any woman look attractive regardless of how much she weighs or what she looks like. It's confidence, not a tiny waist and a big bust that makes a woman look sexy, and by working on your self-esteem and body image you can build your confidence. So stop trying to change the way you look and start changing the way you feel about how you look. Taking the following small steps to a more positive body image can slowly help you feel happier about yourself. (If your body image problems are leading you to develop an unhealthy relationship with food, contact the eating disorders support groups listed in the Resource Guide on page 275 for help, support, advice and information.)

Steps to a More Positive Body Image

TRY TO EASE YOUR SYMPTOMS   It goes without saying that the first step has to be to do all you can to ease your symptoms. This will involve visiting your doctor for treatment and following the healthy diet, exercise and lifestyle advice in our PCOS fertility-boosting plan. Exercise is particularly helpful. The buzz you get from having spent time on yourself will make you look and feel good.

TALK ABOUT IT   Try talking about why you feel so uncomfortable with your body with people you trust, such as family and friends or other women with PCOS. Is there something in particular that makes you feel self-conscious or do you feel self-conscious only in certain circumstances? Why do you think your life will be better when you lose weight, have a clear skin or have shiny, healthy hair? Read some celebrity magazines and you'll soon find lots of stories of unhappy thin women with perfect skins and shiny hair. You don't have to look a certain way to feel healthy, happy and energized.

GIVE YOURSELF AN IMAGE CHANGE   Taking some time to think about how you want to look will help you face the world with more confidence. Have an image change. It could be a new haircut or a new wardrobe, or perhaps you want to try a new shade of lipstick or go for colour analysis or seek the advice of a fashion expert to find out what suits you. Steer clear of darker colours if you are feeling low and wear brighter, more cheerful ones. Unusual accessories can focus other people's attention from any problems you think you have with your figure. And don't underestimate the importance of a well-fitted bra; it can do wonders for your figure.

THROW OUT YOUR OLD CLOTHES   Do yourself a favour and throw out your old clothes. Have you got clothes you never wear or clothes that you used to wear but are too small now that you are hoping to fit into? Throw them out. They are a constant reminder that you haven't lost weight. Living in the past is not good for your self-esteem and body image. Give them to someone who can enjoy them.

STAND TALL   Stand tall. Think about your posture. You will feel more confident about your body and more streamlined if you stand, walk and sit properly. Try reminding yourself to sit properly at your desk on the hour every hour – you'll be surprised how quickly you develop better habits. Or try a course in the Alexander technique to realign your posture permanently.

THINK POSITIVELY   It's not how you look but how you feel about the way you look that matters. Think positively about your body. If you had a friend who kept telling you, you were fat and ugly that she wouldn't be your friend for long. Don't tolerate that kind of treatment from yourself either. If you find this hard, take a good long look at yourself in the mirror. At first you'll see all the bits you don't like, but in time you'll also notice the bits you do – an inviting twinkle in your eyes, the seductive curve of your shoulders, a womanly tummy. Start respecting your body. (Also, look again at our natural tips for boosting libido on page 87 of the PCOS fertility-boosting action plan.)

Step Two: Strengthening Your Relationship With Your Partner

Your relationship with your partner can also come under intense strain during the PCOS fertility rollercoaster. Many women with PCOS talk about the huge burden it places on a relationship if there is difficulty conceiving or they end up not having children. Other women say how hard it is to get in the mood for sex when the weight piles on or when acne, facial hair and absent periods make them feel less feminine. Fertility drugs can also take their toll, and having sex because your doctor says you have to can dampen any couple's enthusiasm.

If you feel that PCOS, anxiety about your fertility and/or fertility treatments are negatively affecting your sex life, then it is important that you get to the root of the problem. First of all, your sex life could simply be affected by a busy life, stress at work and financial worries. Sorting out these problems can lend your relationship a new lease of life.

Take Time to Talk

The problem could simply be that you have stopped talking to each other about how you feel. 'With increasing honesty as you voice your feelings,' says relationship expert and author Steve Biddulph, 'a couple can begin to understand and clear up obstacles to closeness one by one. Love grows through the vulnerability you show, as well as the strength of feelings you admit to.' Try making a pact for a week that, as soon as you see each other at the end of the day, no matter how late it is, you will talk for 10 minutes about the kind of day you had and then for 10 minutes about how the day and/or how the fertility treatment affected you emotionally. This way you give each other support, and build up intimacy, which can otherwise get lost.

Your Sex Life

It can be embarrassing to talk about sex, especially if it hasn't been happening or you aren't enjoying it, so how do you start a conversation? It helps to make the issue a shared one by asking your partner what he thinks or asking how he feels about your sex life. Admit you find it embarrassing but the relationship means a lot to you and you want to start talking. And once you've got the issue out in the open, don't suddenly feel that you have to have mad, passionate sex all the time. It's important that you don't feel under pressure to perform because you have laid your sex life on the line.

Put the emphasis on romance, not on sex. Spending more time together as a couple, whether it's a jog together in the morning or a picnic in the park, a candlelit bath or an evening meal together, can help bring you closer together so you start seeing yourself as lovers again. Try not to neglect the importance of fun. Remember, sex is supposed to be fun, not a battleground. Try things together that you haven't done before. Share jokes, do something a little crazy – like having a dance in the rain – it doesn't matter as long as it's harmless and makes you both laugh.

Perhaps your relationship and your sex life has got into a rut because it's started to seem functional rather than a fun and spontaneous expression of your love and desire for each other as a couple:

> *'I don't think of pleasure anymore when I'm having sex. I think about the drugs I'm taking, the timing, my next doctor's appointment and how much I want to have a baby. My husband feels under pressure and that doesn't help either of us – he once said he feels like a sperm bank and nothing more.'* **PAT, 40**

Try breaking out of this view of sex by focusing on it as a pleasure and a bonding experience for you as a couple. Try adding some variety into your daily and nightly routines. Get up earlier, eat new kinds of food, experiment with different sexual positions and have sex at different times and in different places. Don't wait until you feel good about yourself to be a bit more daring – have a go now. Doing new things and taking risks in and out of bed can make you feel more alive and more attractive.

Physical symptoms of PCOS can also take their toll on your desire to be intimate. If you don't see yourself as a sexual being any more, rediscover your passionate, sexy side by spending time on yourself. Some women find masturbation helpful when they are not having a particularly sexy time in their relationship. If you feel self-conscious about your weight, acne or body hair, buy some sexy underwear, borrow some new perfume or have a facial or a tummy wax.

Plan Some Romance

It may help to plan romance a little more. Plan a time when you and your partner know that you will be alone together. This doesn't always mean you will have sex – it means that you will share intimate moments together. You might end up taking a walk, or cuddling in front of the television. In that special time many things may spontaneously happen and one of them might be sex. Perhaps by midweek you and your partner can agree that on a Saturday you will spend a romantic evening together. By planning, you can set aside time on Saturday to concentrate on feeling your best. You could try something fairly extreme, like getting a new hair style at your hairdresser, or something simple like getting in a nice nap on Saturday afternoon so you don't feel tired by the evening. You want to look forward to some romance and sex, not feel as if it's hard work.

Show Some Affection

And if you aren't in the mood because you feel anxious or worried or tired, instead of withdrawing from intimacy why not initiate it. Don't shut your partner out, hold hands or ask for a hug instead. Make an effort to show physical affection and then receive it when it is given. You'll be surprised how supported, accepted and lovable it makes you feel.

Above all, if you are finding that sex is a problem, don't ignore it. Sex is an important part of a committed relationship. Use books or therapists or videos or whatever works best for you to help your sexual relationship (see also our advice on page 87 in Chapter Two). Don't just ignore it – any good relationship is worth the work.

The gratitude attitude

Feeling and expressing gratitude for the little things your partner does for you can boost the romance in long term relationships, says a study published in the journal *Personal Relationships*. Lead author Dr Sara Algoe, who studied over 65 couples, suggested events such as one partner planning a celebratory meal when the other partner gets a promotion,[254] or stopping to pick up the other partner's favorite coffee drink are each examples of gratuitous behavior that could strengthen romantic relationships, if the recipient feels grateful in response.

The researchers tracked the day-to-day fluctuations in relationship satisfaction and connection for each member of the relationship. These little everyday ups and downs in relationship quality were reliably marked by one person's feelings of gratitude. The effects on the relationship were noticed even the day after feeling the gratitude was expressed. This research thus suggests that even everyday gratitude serves an important relationship maintenance mechanism in close relationships, acting as a booster shot to the relationship.

REMEMBER, THIS ISN'T YOUR FAULT!

If PCOS is the reason you aren't getting pregnant, it can be hard for you not to blame yourself or feel betrayed by your body. You may also feel anxious that your partner will somehow feel let down.

> 'I feel so guilty. I've got it all – a lovely husband, a great job and a good life, but I can't do the one thing that would make our lives perfect – get pregnant. Simon reassures me that he loves me whether or not we have kids but a part of me feels that I have let him down. He loves kids, you see, and would make a fantastic dad. If we don't have kids will he one day turn against me? I'm scared of that and I sometimes think that it would be better for him if he was with someone who could give him kids.'
> CHLOE, 32

This sounds harsh, but having children to fill a hole in your relationship or to make your partner happy is no reason to have children. If your partner feels let down or disappointed or angry this is understandable, but if your relationship is strong enough you will work it through. If you can't work it through then was your relationship strong enough in the first place?

Let Your Partner Support You
A relationship is about loving someone for who they are and taking on board their problems. Turn the tables around. If your partner had a low sperm count would you reject him? No, of course you wouldn't because you love him. So expect the same kind of devotion from your partner. Don't retreat into yourself and push him away. PCOS isn't something you should fight on your own. Let your partner help and support you so you can make decisions about your PCOS and fertility treatment together. This can help you discover whether you really have the right support

in your relationship. Better to discover this now than when you're six months pregnant.

Talking about your relationship and your sex life can help you work out how your partner feels about PCOS and how it and the fertility treatments are affecting things. Without realizing it, you may be unconsciously pushing him away. You might be convinced that your partner is disappointed in you because you aren't fertile, or has stopped fancying you because of PCOS symptoms like weight gain and acne, only to find that they want to help and get close to you again but don't know how to go about it.

Try not to withdraw from your partner at this crucial time in your relationship for fear that he might say things you don't want to hear. At all times include him in the process. This isn't all about you – it's about you and your partner and you need to understand how your partner feels as he's trying to have a baby too and wants to help you stop feeling terrible about yourself if it isn't happening. Initiating discussions and exploring your feelings together about why you can't get pregnant or why you're spending money on fertility treatment can help you discover how much PCOS affects your relationship together. It can also help you find out whether or not your relationship is really ready for a child. Above all, stop blaming yourself if PCOS is making it hard for you to get pregnant. Sure there are things you can do, such as healthy eating and regular exercise, to ease your PCOS symptoms but at the end of the day it remains a condition that for some reason you are susceptible to. 'We don't know enough about PCOS yet to have all the answers,' says Adam Balen, 'but we do know for sure that it isn't your fault if you have it.'

Step Three: Ease Emotional Stress

Just thinking about having a baby can be stressful. Even while you're using ovulation kits you may be worrying about whether you'll be able to handle the 24-hour responsibility of a baby and, as we saw above, trying to make this decision can be one of the first major stresses.

'The stressful nature of trying for a baby with or without fertility treatment is now recognized by experts the world over,' says Harvard infertility specialist Alice Domar. Having a good cry can help you let go of pent up stress, as can talking to your partner or other women with PCOS, but learning how to manage feelings of stress and tension so you don't get so many bad days is even better.

Incorporating the following stress management habits into your life can help you avoid many of the tensions and distresses associated with baby making. If you want to protect your relationship and the health and wellbeing of yourself and your partner and increase your chances of getting pregnant – remember, stress has a negative effect on fertility – we suggest the following:

Continue Your Eating and Exercise Plan
Carry on with the PCOS healthy eating and exercise plan outlined in Chapter Two. Physical wellbeing is an important part of controlling stress. Lack of exercise can also make you feel restless and anxious, so get active. Even simple walking is a great stress reliever. Add it to your routine.

Nurture Yourself
Nurture yourself with relaxation techniques, such as deep breathing from the abdomen, not the chest; meditation; prayer; guided imagery, or yoga. Or simply zone out and daydream every so often. Allow your mind to wander for five minutes every time you feel tense. Maybe use a favourite picture or holiday memory to help you daydream, or find places you know make you feel relaxed and spend some time there as often as you can, even if it's only for 10 minutes in the park at lunchtime.

Be Good to Yourself

Be good to yourself. In scientific studies feeling pleasure, particularly when it involved our senses, has been found to enhance not only our feelings of wellbeing but our health too. For example, gazing at an attractive aquarium of handsome tropical fish was found not only to be relaxing but it lowered blood pressure too. Music, pleasant aromas, and the tastes of certain foods have also been used successfully to relax people and reduce pain, depression and stress.

Think hard about what would give you pleasure. It doesn't have to be anything expensive – you can treat yourself to a bunch of flowers, a manicure or a new mystery novel. Have a long soak in the bath, preferably with a wonderful bath oil or aromatherapy scent – classic essential oils to reduce stress include geranium, lavender, neroli and Roman chamomile. Spend some time by yourself. Get together with women whose lives are not centred around children. Join a book club. Window shop. Go canoeing with your partner. Watch more movies. Spend a weekend in the country and forget what time of the month it is. Whatever you enjoy, think of it as a doctor's prescription for your health and do it regularly.

Practise Mindfulness

Mindfulness is the technique of living here and now and enjoying the present moment. One of the peculiar effects of infertility is that it tends to be so totally absorbing. Your concentration is on what the next step is in your treatment, on what your ovulation kit will show next week, whether you dare to travel next month, whether you had enough sex when you ovulated and so on. Soon there is no room in your mind for what is actually going on around you. By being mindful, by concentrating on every aspect of what you are doing, such as the lunch you're eating, walking down a street, or completing a task, you are both relaxing and nurturing yourself. Your feelings of being stressed out vanish as you focus on finding pleasure in the present moment.

What activity you choose doesn't matter – it can be as simple as peeling an orange or apple – what does matter is your awareness as you go about it. Take your time, peel it slowly, notice the fragrance and colour of the fruit, and pay attention to how it tastes. Remember that the purpose of mindfulness is the deliberate cultivation of your awareness of the here and now. You can take a walk, eat a meal or make love mindfully. The key is to slow down and engage all your senses in what you are doing. Don't worry if your mind wanders – this is entirely normal – learn to watch each thought as it comes and goes. Don't fight wandering thoughts, just be aware of them and then gently turn your attention back to the task in hand.

Express Your Emotions

Not surprisingly, anger is one of the strongest feelings women with PCOS often have. You can feel angry with your body for betraying you, angry at other people for not understanding, angry with the constant waiting, angry with women who do have kids, because it seems so unfair. Expressing your emotions in a journal – even if just for 10 minutes a day – can help you come to terms with much of the negative burden you may not even realize you are carrying. And don't limit yourself to angry emotions – use your journal to write down all your feelings, your grief, your fear, your hope, your disgust, and your self-discovery. You may well find that you gain fresh insights into your emotions and your stress.

Join a PCOS Support Group

Find or form a support group of women with PCOS who are experiencing infertility, whether in your local area or through email or the internet. If infertility is causing you severe anxiety, ask your doctor for help or search for professional counselling. And if infertility is causing severe problems in your relationship, consider joint therapy with a counsellor who specializes in treating infertile couples. If your partner won't join you, go alone.

Step Four: Finding Support

If you're trying for a baby, obviously you'll rely on your partner as a huge source of support and backup. They will know very well what you have gone through in trying to deal with PCOS-related symptoms and the best way to make sure you both aren't overwhelmed is to be upfront about your feelings and share what you are going through. In addition to your partner, it's also important to gather a network of support. If you haven't got a partner and are coping alone, a network of support is absolutely crucial to help you deal with the emotional side of PCOS and fertility treatment. Obviously you have your doctor and fertility specialist to share medical issues with. Partners, family members and friends can also support you by learning more about PCOS, attending support group meetings or doctors' appointments with you and asking what they can do to help. Perhaps your mum knows just the thing that will cheer you up, or your sister knows how to help you stick to a healthy diet. Your close friends can help motivate you to keep fit. Tell them why exercise is important for your health and wellbeing, educate them about PCOS and good friends will be there for you.

Difficulties with Family

Support from the people who care about you is simply the best but unfortunately support from family and friends may not always come automatically – especially if they don't have or don't know anything about PCOS, or have kids already and have never struggled or worried about getting pregnant, or if they live far away, or if you're not comfortable sharing with them.

Dealing with family can be difficult if you are expected to turn up to celebrations where children are present and there will be times when you just can't deal with this.

> 'Christmas has always been hard for Simon and me,' says RACHEL, NOW 44. 'Two years ago we both came back in tears. I took and failed a pregnancy test on Christmas Eve and then had to join in the celebrations. We felt envious of their joy and seeing the children open their presents. In the New Year I told my mum why I wasn't getting pregnant but I wish I hadn't. She just keeps giving me pearls of wisdom that makes things worse, like, "You've got plenty of time" or "Relax and it will happen". She doesn't understand.'

Difficulties with Friends

Things can be just as hard as far as friends are concerned. 'Every one,' says Sally 'and I mean every one of my friends has children now.' If this is the case you could feel you've become the odd one out. It's a lonely feeling and it's happening just when you really need to talk to someone. As months pass and you're still not pregnant you may be surprised at how angry and jealous you feel when you see someone who is pregnant or who has a baby, or if you just hear about someone who has got pregnant. And because you are of childbearing age you are likely to be surrounded by evidence of others' fertility.

It's not uncommon for women with PCOS fertility problems to withdraw from their social lives even to the point where they cease to chat on the phone with anyone who has a child. As a result they feel more isolated and different than ever from people who were once a part of their support system.

> *'I have found it so hard to stay in touch with and share the lives of several of my once good friends,' says* Sue, 36. *'Every time I see their kids I feel annoyed and jealous – and for some reason they can't seem to talk about anything else because their whole lives revolve around their families now. Getting them to organize a babysitter and come out for a girly night is such hard work it makes me feel like I'm imposing. And anyway, I know at some point they'll want to chat about how I'm getting on with trying to get pregnant and be supportive, when really I want them just to take my mind off it for once.'*

Difficulties at Work

It can also be hard to know whether to tell work colleagues or not. If you tell them they may jump to the wrong conclusions and put your career on hold, thinking that you may get pregnant at any moment, not to mention the inevitable 'Are you pregnant yet?' questions. But if you don't tell them, what are you going to say when you need to take time off for tests and appointments? If you don't tell anyone you could come under even more stress as you invent reasons for your absences.

What Can You Do?

So how do you deal with your own expectations and those of others, when you're riding the PCOS fertility rollercoaster?

> *'You need to find the people you can trust who you want to share your emotions, feelings and stresses with,' says* Dominique, 35, *who is currently pregnant with her first child. 'When we first decided to try for a baby, I*

decided I wanted to tell my closest friend about my fears because of PCOS but that I didn't want to tell other friends so I could just go out and feel "normal" when I was with them. But after over a year of trying with no success, I widened my circle of confidantes to include a couple more friends and a colleague at work who had confided in me that she was finding it hard to get pregnant too. That way it wasn't always my husband I was letting off steam with, and I got to turn off the pressure of the stress.'

'I'd say to anyone coping with the PCOS fertility question that you find your own time to tell people,' says KERRI, 42, *who now has two children. 'But that swallowing your pride and asking for support can often be the best thing you can do. I found it hard because first of all I had to explain what PCOS was to several of my friends and my three sisters. But once I had explained it they were so good – and in fact it turned out that the sister I had never been really close to also had PCOS, but hadn't ever told me. So we ended up supporting each other in a really unexpected way.'*

Talking to loved ones, friends and colleagues and explaining the frustrations you are going through with PCOS and your fertility treatment can really help. People aren't mind readers. Unless you explain to them what is going on they can't help or support you. Never underestimate how much people around you do want to listen, understand and be there for you, or how much you will need them to be.

So help yourself and your partner through the rough times by gathering together your own support network, whether friends or family members. If you can't do this or worse still have begun to stay away from family and friends, have no one to talk about your feelings, feel abnormal because you don't have a child and are unable to talk about it with your partner, it is time to seek support from outside help.

PCOS SUPPORT GROUPS   Support can come ready-made in the form of a PCOS support group (see Resource Guide on page 275) where contacts, group meetings, advice, websites, e-mail chat rooms and information for women trying to conceive will be available. 'The emotional support from other women who have PCOS and fertility issues is invaluable,' explains Kristin, 33. 'Peer support offers the ability to talk freely about the issues you have been dealing with. It can be especially wonderful to talk with others who have first-hand knowledge of what you're going through.'

HOSPITAL SUPPORT GROUPS   Check also your local hospital for fertility problems support groups. Many hospitals have informative support groups and, although you may not find so many women with PCOS as you would with a PCOS support group, you'll meet up with couples and other women who are also struggling to have a baby.

Whatever your personal situation, support groups are out there. Even if you feel you want to cope with PCOS and/or fertility treatment alone, the sense of security you can get from knowing there are people you can turn to in times of disappointment, uncertainty and crisis is a huge comfort.

STOP EXPLAINING   The important thing is to get beyond feeling that you need to explain yourself to anyone else and spend some time managing your condition and de-stressing instead. Of course it's up to you how upfront you are with other people, but remember the more people know about PCOS and how it impacts your fertility the less explaining you'll need to do – and the less explaining the millions of other women with PCOS concerned about their fertility, and/or going through fertility treatment, will need to do as well.

Chapter Eight
. . . .
Coming to Terms with Loss and Moving Forward

If you reach a point where you decide that having children isn't going to happen for you, it can be a shock. But it's a sad fact that while many women with PCOS are able to have children eventually, many women experience miscarriage along the way and some women have finally to cope with their inability to have children.

You will need lots of space and time and support to accept that you now need to move to a different path and find a new set of values and coping skills. It may be even harder to accept that one day these values will feel fulfilling – although couples who have been through the transition say that it does happen, albeit slowly.

> 'At the time our world came to an end. We were numb with shock and grief but the things we went through have made us stronger – both as individuals and as a couple, and without realizing it we channelled our creativity into other areas of our life – our jobs, our friends and our family. We have survived and our lives didn't stand still – even though we couldn't see that at the time.' STEVE AND MANDY

You're going to feel a whole range of intense emotions. In addition to a huge sense of loss and pain you may feel as if you have failed. You may grieve that your genes will not continue or that your creativity, so deeply connected to your sexuality, seems to be blocked. You may feel as if you have lost your female identity, and your inability to experience motherhood isolates you from other women. You may feel guilty about previous lifestyle choices to abort or postpone a baby, or angry that you didn't seek help for PCOS earlier.

'Every time I see a mother I feel as if in some way I have failed. I've lost my spark, my zest for life. I hope, I pray, I hope, I curse, I hope and I wish. Some days I feel I don't want to go on if I can't have a baby.' SARAH, 42

'It makes me so angry,' says MARION, 37. *'Even people who have struggled to have kids complain about them. How easily they forget how lucky they are. And those who became parents easily have no idea how lucky they are either!'*

'I feel such pain that I may never have a baby grow inside me. I know I have lots of good things in my life but there is something missing. Why do I long to be a mother? I don't know. All I know is that the future without children looks empty.' LOUISE, 30

'I know lots of women delay having babies because the timing isn't right. But if you've got PCOS you have to be aware that the longer you leave it, the more you reduce your chances compared to women without PCOS. That's what happened to me. I thought I could wait until my late thirties to have a baby but I ended up losing baby after baby. Spending money and time I didn't have on fertility treatment. Nothing worked. The whole business nearly destroyed me. I can't describe the anguish I felt after each miscarriage. The huge sense of sadness, loss and failure that will never leave me. The day I finally decided to stop putting myself through

this monthly torment was a relief, but it was also the bleakest, blackest day of my life.' SUSIE, 42

GIVE YOURSELF PERMISSION TO FEEL

So how on earth do you come to terms with this maelstrom of feelings and get to a stage where you can move on with your life, when suddenly you see babies and pregnant women everywhere and children laughing. All your friends have babies and they belong to a secret world organized around childcare. They look exhausted and stressed but you envy their busy child-full lives and ache with sadness at the empty space in your life.

First of all, you need to let yourself feel, and understand that you're not mad or weak to be feeling like an emotional wreck. The stress on both yourself and your partner can be overwhelming and experts acknowledge that the experience of infertility is hugely traumatic and can make or break a couple. This is because infertility damages self-esteem, triggers many complex emotions and isolates us from the majority of other people. 'In a world that values parenthood,' says US fertility expert Robert Franklin, 'infertile couples feel alone and different; they are often the only couple at the picnic or family reunion without children. Eventually they begin to feel as if they do not belong to this parent-orientated society; they feel abandoned and isolated.'

So before you can move forward, you must say goodbye to your past. You cannot have a baby. Right now, you may find it impossible to gather anything positive from what seems such a black and bitter experience, but if you can look your loss straight in the eye, you will uncover a courage within you. Goodbye isn't easy but grief closes the door behind you so that you can open the door to a new kind of life, and all the opportunities and possibilities that has to offer. These practical steps are suggestions to help you get through the process of grieving and coming to terms with your new life.

LEARN NEW COPING SKILLS

Women struggling with infertility go through a rollercoaster of emotions but one of the biggest concerns is loss of control over their bodies and their lives.

'There is not a single person going through infertility who feels in control,' says London-based infertility psychologist, Sonia Heiger. In addition to loss of control, infertility can also throw your value system into chaos. Most of us are brought up to believe that through hard work you can achieve pretty much anything, that there is justice in the world and that, if you do right, life will treat you right in return. But as we've seen, infertility turns all this on its head. Most childless couples have worked hard to have a baby, lived decent lives and still justice does not prevail.

The values that may have been governing your life until now may not be helping you deal with the experience of infertility so, in order to deal with it and regain a sense of control over your life, you need to learn new coping skills.

LET THE PAST GO

Guilt and pain from the past can reappear and drive the knife of infertility even deeper. A previous abortion, for example, can be one of the most painful memories that you can face and it is hard not to see your current infertility as a punishment. If this is the case, you need to reconsider the circumstances surrounding the abortion and understand that abortion is a loss and must be grieved in order to heal the pain and move forward.

STOP JUDGING YOURSELF BY YOUR FERTILITY

When you can't have a baby, it's because your reproductive process is failing, not because you or your partner are failures. It isn't easy but you need to develop a correct sense of yourself and understand that you are far more than just your ability to conceive. Try not to think that, because fertility is failing, all areas of your life are failing. Having babies is important but, if you are to survive this, you must get it into perspective. 'Try to keep the focus narrow by reminding yourself that only a part of your body is infertile, not your entire being,' says Harriette Rovner-Ferguson, a New York psychotherapist specializing in infertility. For example, she notes that when the late President Ronald Reagan was dealing with a serious medical condition, he put it in perspective when he said, 'my stomach has cancer, I don't.'

Even today, despite all the exciting options that are open to women and all that we can and do achieve, if you can't get pregnant it can be hard not to think of yourself as 'less than'. We still place a high premium on our role as mother and not having children, if you have been conditioned to think that your purpose in life was to have children, can be a crushing blow to your self-worth. 'I've got this huge and amazing career but at times I feel like I haven't really succeeded as a woman,' says Mary. 'It's daft and un-PC but without a child I feel like I haven't achieved that much.' (If this is you, turn to page 223 for our tips on building self-esteem)

MANAGE STRESS POSITIVELY

You need to learn to manage the stress of infertility in a positive way. Healthy eating and regular exercise is a great way to reduce stress, as is talking more with close friends and family and getting involved in infertility support groups. Staying positively focused and reminding yourself that it is your infertility treatment that is failing and not you will help you reframe the experience in a less negative light. If you have difficulty doing this, a professional counsellor or therapist can help you change negative thinking about yourself and your life to a positive, or at least more acceptable, form.

Coping with loss means that you give yourself permission to be angry and to cry. Anger is an important part of grieving and you need to express it to release stress, but it is important to realize that your anger is directed at the problem and not at your kid sister who has just got pregnant, or your boss who's got five kids, or the social worker who visits your house to see if it is suitable for adoption when you know that most people don't have to go through this. Crying is important because grief is the body's natural healer when it comes to emotional loss. At times it may seem too painful, but the only way to heal is to let yourself feel the sorrow without feeling guilty. If you refuse to face the grief it won't heal and you may get stuck in it (see the Five Stages of Grief on page 252).

TAKE CARE OF YOUR PARTNER TOO

Sharing your grief with someone you care about, preferably your partner, is the key to releasing bottled-up tension. When you and your partner share your grief you can grow closer, because it is by communicating your vulnerability that you lay the grounds of intimacy. This doesn't mean the hurt disappears, it means that the bond of understanding and affection grows. Problems tend to occur when one partner feels isolated from the other, but couples need to understand that infertility is a 'we' problem, not a 'my' problem. 'Although many marriages are strengthened during an infertility work up, the divorce rate is high among infertile couples, especially those who are unable to share their feelings,' says Dr Franklin, Professor of Gynecology at Baylor College of Medicine in Houston, Texas. So it is important to reach out to your partner, and protect your relationship, as he is likely to be feeling as vulnerable and as hurt as you are right now. Infertility doesn't have to do permanent damage to your union. The crisis can be a learning opportunity – a chance to learn more about your partner's coping style as well as a time to learn more about how to take care of each other.

ACCEPT THAT MEN COPE DIFFERENTLY

Men and women are different in many ways. Men are often more problem-solving while women tend to vent their feelings, and expecting your partner to mirror your coping skills can be disappointing.

> 'I just wanted someone to hold me and listen and say, "Yes, it must be awful, you must feel terrible and I sympathize," but my partner wouldn't want to hold to that sense of grief or "wallow in it", as he put it. He would say, "OK, if we can do this, do that, try again, we can have a baby next time." He meant well in trying to be positive, but at the time I just needed someone to acknowledge the depths of my hurt.' EMMA, 33

You may not get all that you need from your partner and a better option may be to supplement his support with that you receive from your friends and family.

HONE YOUR COMMUNICATION SKILLS

In order to cope with infertility you need good communication skills. You need to let your partner and the people close to you know how you want to be treated. Infertile women often communicate what the problem is but they don't always let their listeners know what they feel and what they need. For example, compare, 'I've had a pregnancy test and I'm not pregnant,' with, 'I've had a pregnancy test today and I'm not pregnant. I feel miserable and hopeless and need to be held.' The latter message is more likely to be understood because the entire message is communicated, whereas the first leaves the listener uncertain what to do to help.

JOIN A SUPPORT GROUP

At whatever stage you are in your fertility treatment, whether waiting for results, grieving or deciding to withdraw or considering adoption, it is worth thinking about the various infertility support groups that exist both locally and nationally. Not only can they give you advice and information, but they can put you in touch with other people going through what you are going through. They also have numerous helplines for particular issues and experiences. You may find that you get all you need from a PCOS support group or that infertility organizations are more tailor-made to your needs. Most but not all clinics also have patient support groups which can provide information, leaflets and addresses and activities. You may find the idea of joining a group scary or depressing, as it acknowledges you have a problem, but you don't have to go to meetings – you can pledge your support by staying in touch via newsletters that are reassuring and comforting, or visiting infertility support web sites and chatrooms (see Resource Guide on page 275 for details).

THE FIVE STAGES OF GRIEF

Since confronting grief can be intensely painful and overwhelming, we often try to protect ourselves by avoiding it, but grief is a normal healing process that has to be experienced in order for us to move forward. The last thing you may want to do is face it but grief is the only way our bodies know how to heal the pain. 'Regardless of whether the grief is real, in response to an actual loss, or anticipated, when a treatment cycle fails, it must be experienced,' says Franklin. 'It is by experiencing our feelings through grief that we help them go away. If we fail to do this they linger, causing us suffering.'

Research has shown that infertile couples need to allow themselves to grieve and to express their anger and anguish. Without such expression the feelings remain unresolved, and the five stages of grief model outlined below has now been applied to infertility counselling. We all grieve in different ways but, regardless of our grieving style, there are predictable stages that we all go through, although not always in the same order. If you're coping with the trauma of infertility, the five stages of grief outlined below are entirely normal and natural.

Stage One: Shock and Denial

The first stage of grief is shock and or denial. Even if you know that you have PCOS and that it can affect your fertility, you might still be stunned to discover that you have a fertility problem. Once you can accept that you have a problem, the diagnosis isn't so painful to hear and you can begin to talk about your problem, seek advice, help and support and move out of this stage of grief.

Stage Two: Anger

Not being able to have children when you want to seems cruelly unfair. It's as if Nature has cheated you of your birthright and you may well find yourself experiencing the 'why me?' syndrome. 'Why me? When so many women can and often shouldn't have a baby, why can't I get pregnant?' This anger may build into rage when you do everything humanly possible and still no pregnancy occurs. Sometimes that anger may get directed away from 'why me?' into 'why you?', and anyone who reminds you of the fact that you can't get pregnant will become the target of your anger – your partner, your sister with her lovely new baby, your doctor and the pregnant world at large. But by far the most harmful anger is the one that is directed against yourself. You may get so angry with yourself that self-esteem falters, leaving only an overwhelming sense of failure.

Stage Three: Bargaining

Feeling desperate, you may start to bargain with your god or a higher force in order to gain a feeling of control. You may actually believe that, if you are a better person or do this or that good deed, then you'll become pregnant. Sadly, when the good deed doesn't translate into pregnancy, this can make you feel even more out of control and exhausted and abandoned – as if you did your part, but the universe didn't respond.

Stage Four: Feeling Hopeless and Helpless

With every loss or failure of treatment you may begin to feel more and more hopeless and helpless. This is the most vulnerable stage when you could sink into a depression where there is no hope and no positive options. Many couples refer to this stage as the black hole stage. You may experience this month after month, when hopes are dashed by a negative pregnancy test, or you may experience it when you finally decide to call it a day and stop treatment. If this happens, the danger is that you lose your resilience to build up hope again and lack the mental energy to pull yourself through, and professional help may be needed to help you learn effective coping strategies.

Stage Five: Acceptance

The final stage involves accepting that you have a problem and that you may never be able to have a child of your own. This is the stage when you admit that you have a problem and that it hurts – it hurts a lot. Acceptance doesn't mean that your grieving is over but that it's managed in a way that is healthy for you and your partner. Yes, you want a baby but you accept that you can't have one and this isn't your fault. The pain of your loss is a part of your life but it doesn't control your life because you find ways to cope with it. You may be able to do this alone and/or with the support of family and friends, or you may need the support of a counsellor or therapist.

INFERTILITY COUNSELLING

Counselling isn't the same as psychotherapy or psychoanalysis, which assume deep disturbances that have their root in childhood. Counselling starts from the idea of addressing current issues in your life, such as infertility, and exploring painful feelings associated with them. Infertility is a life crisis and your fertility specialist simply won't have the time to help you and your partner take stock of any news that hits you. Counselling provides a quiet space for you and your partner to mull over your feelings and get the support and information you need. We'd urge any couple going through fertility treatment to include counselling as a couple in their treatment plan.

Seeing a counsellor doesn't mean there is anything wrong with you. It just means that infertility is causing you to feel a range of turbulent emotions and you may need to talk these through with someone. In the UK, the HFEA Act states that all people receiving fertility treatment must, before consenting to treatment, be given opportunities to receive proper counselling to help them understand any treatment they are having and to help them adjust their expectations and accept situations.

Professional fertility counsellors are an important part of any fertility clinic. They are medically informed and can help you make decisions about your treatment and cope with the consequences. You are well advised to ask right at the beginning of your relationship with a clinic what their counselling service consists of, and, if it is an added cost, how much it will be. If there is a cost, you may prefer to see your doctor and find out if his or her practice has an in-house counsellor you could see, or you may prefer to find your own counsellor outside the clinic.

There could be reasons why you don't want to go to counselling. You might have your own way of coping and friends and family who can give you all the support you need. That's fine, but we do recommend that you check out your clinic's counsellor to see whether or not you might find it of special benefit.

COPING WITH MISCARRIAGE

Miscarriage is far more common than you may realize, regardless of whether you have PCOS or not. An estimated one in four women experience miscarriage and one in 300 have had three or four miscarriages. But if you experience a miscarriage, you might have been surprised by the enormity of your grief. Like millions of women, from the earliest stages of pregnancy you perhaps recognize the developing fetus as an integral part of yourself.[256] Researchers LG Peppers and RJ Knapp found no differences in the intensity or patterns of grief among women who miscarried or experienced stillbirth or neonatal death.

Your loss may feel so painful because there is an immediate psychological bonding between a mother and her fetus. 'The major changes in a woman's hormonal make up take place early in pregnancy, almost just after conception,' writes Jonathon Scher, MD, author of *Preventing Miscarriage: The Good News*. 'Mothers undergo huge hormonal fluctuations and we tend to think this grows along with her swelling belly. But in fact the greatest impact occurs early in pregnancy. So when you lose a pregnancy, there is scientific (hormonal) proof that these feelings occur."

In an attempt to avoid the pain, many women struggle not to grieve over a miscarriage, but as we stressed earlier, when you are coming to terms with the failure of treatment, it is vital for emotional recovery and growth to mourn fully such a profound loss. Only when we allow ourselves to feel painful feelings and share our grief with people we trust are we able to begin the healing process.

If you have miscarried, even if it was early on, it can be tempting to rush ahead with the next treatment cycle. However, miscarriage is a big deal and you need to treat it with the respect you and your unborn baby deserve. It is crucial that you are kind and nurturing towards yourself at this time and avoid any situations, such as baby showers, that are going to cause pain. Give yourself the time and the space to grieve and to accept and experience all your feelings.

Grief isn't something you can run away from. Symptoms of grief have been observed in women 20 years after their miscarriage.[257] Don't be surprised if you feel a huge sense of guilt and self-blame and worry that you miscarried because of something you did, like riding a bike or eating strawberries. It can't be stressed enough that miscarriage is not your fault but, when you are in pain and desperate to find answers, you may well blame yourself or even your doctor or fertility clinic.

Freeing yourself from such negative feelings can add to your sense of closure and may well also contribute to the success of future treatments, if you decide that is what you want to do. In a study of 195 couples with a history of recurring miscarriage, researchers found that, among women who were involved in emotional recovery programmes, 85 percent conceived again, while of those in the control group only 35 percent had successful pregnancies.[258] What's more, if you have unresolved grief, this may stop you fully experiencing the joy of any future pregnancy.

Healing Self-Blame Visualization

Sit comfortably and close your eyes. Breathe deeply and release what tension you can. Imagine a bright light shining on you and sucking out any tension that is left, and the only weight that is left is a bag you have on your back that the light cannot penetrate. This bag is filled with self-blame and anger. Feel the weight of the bag as you walk towards the ocean. Take the bag off your back, open it and pull out the blaming words and phrases, which you repeat aloud and throw them one by one into the ocean – hurl them like heavy stones into the sea. Watch the tide carry your self-blame away and walk away, feeling stronger and lighter with every step.

'If you feel that you have not fully grieved over a miscarriage,' says Niravi Payne, founder of the Whole Person Fertility Program in New York, 'I recommend that you express what you are feeling – verbally or nonverbally – by engaging in some form of grief ceremony.' This can be a funeral or you may also want to write a letter to your unborn child or say a prayer, or record your experiences in a diary. The important thing is to acknowledge your grief.

SECONDARY INFERTILITY

'People would keep telling me every time a treatment failed, "Never mind, you have a child." And I would just say to people, "Look I don't want to be reassured, I just want to tell you that I know I have a lovely daughter already but I want another child so badly."' Sylvia, **38**

If you've got pregnant once, this isn't always a guarantee that you will get pregnant again, especially if PCOS is the case and your chances of conceiving are less than women without. Secondary infertility is not as rare as it sounds and the condition is even more common statistically than primary infertility. According to the National Center for Health Statistics, more than half of American women who could not conceive or carry a child to term already had at least one child. Other estimates are as high as 70 percent.

Couples with secondary infertility are often assumed to be fertile because they have a child and, as a result, they are only half as likely to seek out medical treatment. But if you want another child and have PCOS, don't assume that second time round will not be a problem. It isn't a good idea to delay treatment, as we've seen how PCOS can negatively impact your fertility.

The Links with PCOS

Why is PCOS linked to secondary infertility? If you've put on rather than lost baby weight from last time, can this make your symptoms worse? Or is it because you're a stressed working mum and it's put you under strain? The feelings of couples unable to have more than one child are often slighted, and, if this is your situation, you may find that your position invokes jealousy rather than solidarity with those who are childfree. Since you have a child already, people tend to feel that your disappointment isn't so great. This simply isn't the case. 'Secondary infertility hurts. You may be surprised how much. You probably never anticipated that the inability to complete your desired family could cause such pain,' says Massachusetts infertility therapist and support group leader for RESOLVE, Harriet Fishman Simons. 'The sense of failure and anguish is just as deep as for the woman who never gives birth, because they feel the loss of their dream of a larger family.'

'I've always dreamed of having four children, a couple of dogs and a house with a large garden for the kids to play in. That dream might never come true now and my throat hurts and my eyes well with tears whenever I think of it.' MARINA, 39

Treatment for secondary infertility would be no different than for primary infertility and therapy for secondary infertility should also be along the same lines. It involves acknowledging the grief, managing stress productively, learning new coping skills and gathering support.

A DIFFERENT LIFE

You may not be able to see it at the moment but there are compensations to being childfree. When you feel ready, you can begin to concentrate on these advantages, the most significant being your freedom – freedom to pursue your interests, career or vocation, and freedom to live your life the way you choose. Perhaps you will travel, perhaps you will work with children in another capacity, perhaps you will find other ways to mother. You can mother or nurture other people, siblings, friends, parents, ideas, communities, projects, jobs, plants, animals and so on. Whatever you decide nothing will be as tough as the endless cliffhanger of infertility treatment.

'There are infinitely more ways to lead a meaningful, successful life than by becoming a parent,' says family therapist Beverly Engel, who practises in Cambria, California. 'Childfree living need not be merely tolerated but can be a positive, fulfilling and joyous experience.'

Not being able to have your own children doesn't mean you can't include children in your life. You can make an incredible impact on their lives by teaching, mentoring and role modelling. There are opportunities to befriend and tutor children, sponsor a child in another country, work with children in a professional and voluntary capacity, become a mentor, act as godparent or caretaker for your friend's and family's children, and so on. There are so many contributions to make to a child's development. You don't have to look far to find a child who can benefit from some of your time and attention, and you should never underestimate the impact that this can have on the life of a child. It is high time that we begin to value these contributions as highly as the birthing experience.

> 'I look back now to the anguish of every month, when periods arrived without any respect for my feelings, and my overwhelming desire to be a Mom and I can't believe we got through it and came out the other side. We finally made the decision not to put ourselves through this any more after a lot of talking with each other and with my PCOS sisters online. It still hurts to think we can't have kids that will share our genetic heritage – but I can bring all my mothering skills, and Don can bring all of his fathering skills into the lives of our nieces and nephews, and the kids at the playgroup where I finally got the courage to work. It's a different way to be a Mom but I'm getting so much out of it.' DIONNE, 42

Shaping a successful social life can be hard if you are surrounded by people with children and many friends drift apart when one has children and the other doesn't. If this is the case and common ground can't be found between you, then you need to seek out friends who are also child- free. Seek out those who are living happy and positive childfree lives and get to know them. In order to do that, you need to get involved in activities that are not child-centred such as discussion groups, travel clubs and so on. Let people know you are looking to hook up with other childfree people – you'll find lots of them and there is no need to feel alone. The number of childfree women is increasing every year and the

US now has a childfree network with over 50 places for childfree people and, in the UK, ISSUE has set up an organization for childfree people called More to Life (see Resource Guide on page 275 for details).

BRINGING CHILDREN INTO YOUR LIFE

If you feel you want to experience mothering, even though you can't carry a child yourself, and you and your partner agree that this is something you want to look at, adoption and fostering can offer you the chance to raise kids.

Adoption

> *'I don't think I could have got through this whole PCOS infertility nightmare without the knowledge that adoption was a possibility. We just felt we had so much love to give and after six years of infertility treatment we began to accept that maybe our role was to give that love in another way. I had to work hard and fight every inch of the way but eventually we became the proud parents of our, and "our" in every sense of the word, adopted sons. From the moment I saw them at five months old they were my babies – my long awaited children.'* ANNA, 34

Should you be considering adoption, you will find that you need to go through a barrage of assessments that can be daunting and stressful and frustrating. Most adoption agencies will only consider your application if you have given up fertility treatment entirely. The main reason is to ensure that the couple have come to terms with their infertility.

Adoption agencies expect both partners to be in reasonably good health. Your social background will be taken into account. Most will look at your income and you will need to demonstrate that you can care materially for a child. Adoption demands great commitment from you and your partner and you both need to appear committed and positive in front of everyone involved with the adoption. It can be tough, and time consuming – but then, so can fertility treatment, and if you really want to give a child a warm, loving home, it's worth looking into this option.

Research has shown that contrary to people's fears, adopted children turn out to be well-adjusted and stable as well as normally intelligent. 'Obviously all parents – both fertile and infertile – worry about how their children will develop,' says fertility expert Robert Winston. 'There is not the slightest evidence that adopted children are worse off.'

Your adopted child will have the right and the need to know that he or she is adopted and you must be ready to deal with your child's need to discover their past at some point in the future. This should not create long-term difficulties as it is the nurturing aspect of parenthood that impacts a child far more than the biological. If they do want to make contact, their curiosity is natural and does not reflect on the adopting parents and the relationship that they have built up with the child.

If you think you would like to adopt a child, the first thing to do is to contact your nearest adoption agency (see Resource Guide on page 275 for details). You've got the best chance if you're in a relationship and aged between 21 and 35 (40 for the man), but, because of the surplus of children with special needs, these rules will become far more flexible in these cases and there are opportunities for single women and older couples to put their case forward.

There are no guarantees that you will be matched with a child and, even when it does all fall into place, it's still hard work that's never going to go away. Adoption isn't for everyone. It has its challenges as well as its joys and not every couple will feel emotionally equipped to deal with it, but if you do decide to adopt, it could turn out to be one of the best decisions you ever made.

Fostering

In many ways fostering is no different from adoption. You take care of a child's emotional, physical, social and educational needs on a daily basis. The only difference is that, when you foster a child, you don't become their legal parents and may also share their care with their birth parents.

Children who need foster care are those who, for whatever reason, are vulnerable in their home environment. The family unit may have broken down or there may be learning difficulties or disability. Whatever the reason, the birth parents are in crisis and can't cope alone. The Local Authority steps in and helps the family sort out its problems and develop strategies for the child's future.

Applying to become a foster carer does involve a lot of paperwork and assessment by social workers. You might have to undergo a short period of training as it is likely that many of the children put up for foster care will be troubled or confused.

Foster carers can feel powerless since they have few legal rights over the child. They may also be vulnerable to allegations of abuse, since many of the children they are caring for will be emotionally damaged. You may long to bond with your foster child but at the end of the day you know that they can at any minute be returned to their real parents, and this may stop you becoming too attached. So fostering does require great strength of mind, stamina and compassion. (For more information see our Resource Guide on page 275.)

Mentoring

In the US there are lots of opportunities to get involved in the lives of children if adoption doesn't work out. You could offer support and inspiration to a disadvantaged child by becoming a mentor, or join the Big

Brothers/Big Sisters of America programme. (Again, see our Resource Guide on page 275.)

FINAL REMINDERS FOR INFERTILE COUPLES

Every couple must find their own way to cope with being childfree but here are some general points which may help if you have PCOS and have been told no further treatment is possible:

Allow Yourself to Mourn
Being told you are infertile is a bitter blow. You may feel that the pain is something you will never get over, but the healing process can only begin when you grieve and really cry. Give yourself the time, the space and the right to mourn. Only when you do that can you begin to deal with the situation and live again.

Stop Worrying About the Past
It doesn't help to think about how you postponed the baby decision too long, or to dwell on an abortion you had that was necessary at the time when your situation was different. Nor does it help to keep remembering the reasons why you didn't seek help for PCOS earlier. You had your reasons and there is no point dwelling on 'what ifs… ?'

Don't Blame Yourself
If PCOS contributed to your infertility, stop feeling guilty or blaming yourself. PCOS is not your fault and it isn't your fault that you can't get pregnant. 'In my experience,' says Robert Winston, 'infertility is never anyone's fault – just as catching influenza or developing cancer is no one's fault.'

Accept You Have Tried Your Best
Accept that you did all that you could. If you don't think you did all that you could, have the courage to face that fact and acknowledge the reasons why.

Don't Let Your Feelings Take Over Your Life
Try not to let your feelings dominate your relationships with friends and family. While it is good to be open with those who care about you, continued reference may be difficult for some of your friends to cope with.

Don't Be Seduced By 'Wonder Treatments'
Infertility treatment sells newspapers, so ignore all those sensational headlines about new treatments or women giving birth in their sixties. Remain healthily skeptical about over-optimistic success rates reported in the press.

Communicate With Your Partner
Your best support is likely to be your partner. Work out how you can spend more times doing things together. See how you can make sex a pleasure again, rather than a baby-making process. Infertility has many destructive effects on relationships but it can also have the positive effect of strengthening and improving it. Do your best to ensure that it enhances the positive aspects of your relationship and your life.

Seek Support
Join a support group for people who are childfree (see Resource Guide on page 275).

Choose Your Language Carefully

Language can be powerful. Therefore it's important that you decide on the term you wish to use for your status regarding children. Some people prefer the term 'childfree' to the term childless because the latter connotes a loss of some sort, incompleteness or deficiency. If you've been trying hard for a baby, you may not feel free at all but you do have an option to live childfree instead of continuing the struggle to have a baby when it was clear it wasn't going to happen. You do have the choice to stop your treatments and experience a different way of life.

Develop Other Parts of Your Life

Ask yourself whether you have the chance to develop other aspects of your life. If you are not bringing up children, you are likely to have more time and more freedom. Perhaps you could put more into your job. Hobbies, your home, friendships, family, travel or voluntary service are other areas where many child-free women find ways to make radical changes in their lives and radical benefits to the lives of others.

Remember All Life Choices Bring Compromise

Try to remember that motherhood, as rewarding and as absorbing as it is, is a phase, like studying for an exam or seeing a big research project through. It does, of course, start a lifelong relationship, but then so does having a best friend, a lover or a brother or sister. Life is about more than bringing up children, and everyone finds this out – even mothers when their children finally leave home – it's just something childfree women learn earlier. Sure, childfree women miss out, but nobody can have everything and mothers miss out too. They spend a good deal of their lives tired, anxious or preoccupied. When one door is closed, no amount of anger or tears will open it, but other doors will open. Why not see what options and possibilities are on the other side?

Afterword
. . . .
Your Onward Journey

You may decide that you want to try for a baby now or some time in the future. You may decide that children are not for you. You may get pregnant easily or you may have to enlist the support of medical technology to achieve the family you want to have. You may decide that adoption or fostering are ways forward for you. You may have to struggle to get the treatment you want and need. Whatever path lies ahead of you, reading about the options and possibilities available will help you feel less vulnerable, more in charge and more informed so that you can make a decision that works for you.

There are three things we hope you'll take away with you from reading this book: the first is that getting informed is the best way to feel more in control, and that as well as this book, talking to your doctor, and other women with PCOS is a great way to find out more.

> 'Trying to get my doctor to give me information was like banging my
> head against a brick wall. But when I found other women over the
> internet who were sharing lots of tips and advice they'd got from their
> doctors or specialists it made me feel much better and less out of control.
> I realized I wasn't infertile full stop, and that there were options like
> Clomid and metformin to help me on my way. That gave me the boost
> I needed to decide I'd have a go at getting pregnant. It took away my

sense of loneliness and fear of the unknown. And after nearly two years of trying on our own and then deciding to get help, the Clomid worked and I'm expecting a bouncing baby.' PATRICIA, 34

'Just finding out from my specialist that many women with PCOS become Moms took the feeling of pressure right out of me. I was told when I first got diagnosed that at 26, I should really be thinking about kids given my condition. And I'm sure my desperation showed through and put off all the guys I was dating! When I finally got the information I needed I felt much more relaxed. I've now got a special someone in my life and, well, I'm finally happy to wait and see what happens next!' SHERIE, 28

The second, is that taking care of yourself is well worth the effort – by making changes to your and your partner's diet and lifestyle you really can make a big difference to your chances of conceiving with PCOS. It might sound really simple but it's really powerful too, and something that's within your control every day.

'My daughter Noa was born in October 2003 after a straighforward pregnancy and natural labour. I followed the PCOS Diet Book guidelines prior to getting pregnant and as much as I could when I was pregnant, and I am sure this helped me to feel great the whole way through. Learning how important diet is when you've got PCOS really focused me on what to do to help myself. Two of my friends with PCOS have also just had babies after making the diet and lifestyle changes.' EVE

'I couldn't believe that seeing a nutritionist could make such a difference to my life! I felt so low, stressed out and depressed about not getting pregnant, and a friend of mine recommended this idea as she had found it had cured her PMS. So I went to find out more about getting my health

back on track by eating well, with a real determination to do something positive for myself after so long doing myself down for "failing". It sounds corny, but nourishing myself with good food and taking time out to see my body as my friend to take care of, not my enemy, gave me a whole new store of energy to try for a baby again. And it gave our relationship a whole new zing because my low moods had lifted and I remembered that being in love with this wonderful man was the reason I wanted to have a baby in the first place. We're trying for our second child now and I'd recommend a self-care programme to anyone.' **HEATHER, 37.**

Finally, asking for support from other women and their partners who are going through PCOS can be a really fantastic experience – there's nothing quite like being able to chat or email with someone who knows what you're going through – and might even have a few tried and tested ideas to help you through your PCOS fertility journey.

'The hardest thing for me about having PCOS is thinking about whether I want to have kids or not. At the moment I just don't know and I really don't want PCOS to make me panic. I'd say to every woman out there in the same situation that I am, talk to each other through support groups, and talk to your husbands and your families – the more talking you do the clearer it gets.' **GABY, 31.**

And knowing how much help it can be to get that support, we'd love to ask you to try and offer it too, if you're ever in a position where you can. After all, the more women with PCOS who ask questions, share stories and talk about what has worked for them to boost fertility, the more we'll have to contribute when we see our doctors and specialists, and the better treatment we – and the women who come after us – will get. And every little helps – just posting your story on a support group website anonymously will ring bells with someone out there who's been feeling what you've been feeling, and wishing someone else knew what it was like. You really can touch the lives of other women going through their PCOS fertility journeys, as well as taking charge of your own.

We hope this book has helped you on your way.

Resource Guide
Useful Contacts

If you want to find out more about PCOS in general, or hook up with other women dealing with fertility issues, or find out more about women's fertility, these are some of the best and most relevant contacts, books and websites. Remember, the beauty of websites is that they are international, so you can get some great help and information from any of the websites listed here, not just from organizations, based in your country. If you do write to an organization always send a stamped addressed envelope, as many of these places are charities and run by volunteers.

In addition to your doctor's advice, a PCOS support group should be your first port of call. Groups like Verity in the UK or PCOS Support in the US can help put you in touch with a support group in your area and also give you the advice, help and information that you need to make informed choices about PCOS and your fertility.

UNITED KINGDOM

PCOS

Verity

The Graystone Centre
28 Charles Square
London N1 6HT
www.verity-pcos.org.uk

Adoption and Fostering

Adoption Information Line

193 Market Street
Hyde SK14 1HF
0800 793 4086
www.adoption.org.uk

British Agencies for Adoption and Fostering (BAAF)

Skyline House
200 Union Street
London SE1 0LX
020 7593 2000
www.baaf.org.uk

Adoption UK – Advice and Support

Manor Farm
Appletree Road
Chipping Warden
Banbury OX17 1LH

0870 7700 450
www.adoptionuk.org

National Foster Care Association (NFCA)

Leonard House
517 Marshalsea Road
London SE1 1EP
020 7357 8015
www.epolitix.com

Overseas Adoption Helpline

First Floor, 34 Upper Street
London N1 0PN
020 7226 7666

Gay and Lesbian Foster Carers Association

c/o London Friend
86 Caledonian Road
London N1 9DN
020 8854 8888 x2088

Biological Clock Anxiety

British Association for Counselling

1 Regent Place
Rugby CV21 2PJ
01788 550899/578328
www.bac.co.uk

Exploring Parenthood
4 Ivory Place
Treadgold Street
London W11 4BP
020 7221 6681

Family Planning Association
2–12 Pentonville Road
London N1 9FP
020 7837 5432
www.fpa.org.uk

Relationship Guidance

Relate
Herbert Gray College
Little Church Street
Rugby CV21 3AP
01788 573241
www.relate.org.uk

Complementary Therapies

Alternative Health Information Bureau
01923 469495

Centre for the Study of Complementary Medicine
01703 334752

British Holistic Medical Association
59 Lansdown Place
Hove BN3 1FL
01273 725951
www.bhma.org.uk

British Complementary Medicine Association
249 Fosse Road
Leicester LE3 1AE
0116 282 5511
www.bcma.uk

National Institute of Medical Herbalists
56 Longbrook Street
Exeter EX4 6AH
01392 426022
www.nimh.org.uk

Register of Chinese Herbal Medicine
020 8904 1357
www.rchm.co.uk

British Homeopathic Association
27a Devonshire Street
London W1N 1RJ
020 7935 2163
www.trusthomeopathy.org

Society of Homeopaths
01604 621400
www.homeopathy-soh.org

British Acupuncture Council
Park House
206–8 Latimer Road
London W10 6RE
020 8735 0400
www.acupuncture.org

British Hypnotherapy Association
020 7723 4443
www.hypnotherapy-uk.org

Aromatherapy Organizations Council
PO Box 355
Croydon CR9 2QP
020 8251 7912
www.aocuk.net

International Federation of
Aromatherapists
020 8742 2605
www.int-fed-aromatherapy.
co.uk

International Federation of
Reflexologists
020 8667 9458

www.reflexology-ifr.com

Association of Reflexologists
27 Old Gloucester Street
London WCIN 3XX
08705 673320
www.aor.org.uk

Transcendental Meditation
Beacon House
Willow Walk, Woodley Park
Skelmersdale WN8 6UR
08705 143733

General Council and Register of
Naturopaths
Frazer House
6 Netherhall Gardens
London NW3 5RR
020 7435 6464
www.naturopathy.org.uk

Her Trust
21J Devonshire Place
London W1G 6HZ
020 7935 9315
www.hertrust.com

Also:
Michelle Roques-O'Neil at
www.purealchemy.co.uk

Reflexologist Jacqui Garnier
at Garnier70@aol.com

Diabetes

British Diabetic Association
10 Queen Anne Street
London W1M 0BD
020 7323 1531
www.diabetes.org.uk

Eating Disorders

Eating Disorders Association
Sackville Place
44, Magdalen Street
Norwich, Norfolk NR3 1JE
0160 362 1414
www.edauk.com

Overeaters Anonymous
01273 624712
Local groups throughout the
UK
www.oagb.org.uk

Fertility and Preconceptual Care

ISSUE: The National Fertility
Association
114 Lichfield Street
Walsall WS1 1SZ

01922 722888
www.issue.co.uk

National Childbirth Trust
Alexander House
Oldham Terrace
London W3 7NH
0870 7703236
www.nct-online.org

Foresight: Association for the
Promotion of Preconceptual Care
28 The Paddock
Godalming GU7 1XD
01483 427839
www.foresight-
preconception.org.uk

Maternity Alliance
Third Floor west
2–6 Northborough Street
London EC1V OAY
0207 490 7638
www.maternityalliance.org.uk

Also:
www.fertilityuk.org
A great fertility website that
promotes fertility awareness
Dr Sarah Temple at www.
privatefamilydoctor.com

Infertility Support

Human Fertilization and Embryo authority (HFEA)
    Paxton House
    30 Artillery Lane
    London E1 7LS
    020 7377 5077
    www.hfea.gov,uk

    (Publishes a patient guide to infertility clinics around the country, with success rates)

CHILD: National Infertility Support Network
    Charter House
    43 St Leonards Road
    Bexhill on Sea TN40 1JA
    01424 732361
    www.child.org.uk

British Infertility Counselling Association
    69 Division Street
    Sheffield S1 4GE
    01342 843880
    www.bica.net

Infertility Support Group
    c/o Women's Health
    52 Featherstone street
    London EC1Y 8RT
    020 7251 6580
    www.womens-health.co.uk/

More-to-Life (UK based childfree network)
    114 Lichfield Street
    Walsall WS1 1SZ
    070 500 37905
    www.moretolife.co.uk

Miscarriage

Miscarriage Association
    c/o Clayton Hospital
    Northgate
    Wakefield WF1 3JS
    01924 200799
    www.miscarriageassociation.
    org.uk

Miscarriage support group listings:
    www.kumc.edu/gec/support/
    miscarri.html

Nutrition

British Association of Nutritional Therapists
    27 Gloucester Street

London WIN 3XX
0870 6061284
www.bant.org.uk

Women's Nutritional Advisory Service
01273 487366
www.wnas.org.uk

Women's Health

Women's Health
52 Featherston Street
London EC1Y 8RT
020 7251 6580
www.womens-health.co.uk/

For information about self-insemination and UK clinics that do not discriminate against single women or lesbians: Rights of Women (same address, 020 7251 6577); Lesbian Parenting (same address, 020 7251 6576)

USA

PCOS

Polycystic Ovarian Syndrome Association Inc (PCOSA)
PO Box 80517
Portland, OR 97280
USA
+877 775 PCOS
www.pcosupport.org

PCOTeen (A division of PCOSA)
www.pcosupport.org/pcoteen/about.html

www.soulcysters.com
Online support and a place to share PCOS histories

Adoption, Fostering and Mentoring

National Council for Adoption
1930 17th Street, NW
Washington, DC 20009
USA
+202 328 1200
www.ncfa-usa.org

National Foster Care Association
    www.nfpainc.org

National Council for Single Adoptive Parents
    PO Box 15084
    Chevy Chase, MD 20815
    USA
    +202 966 6367
    www.adopting.org

Adoptive Families of America, Inc
    2309 Como Avenue
    St Paul, MN 550108
    USA
    +800 372 3300
    www.adoptivefam.org

National American Council on adoptable children
    970 Raymond Avenue, Suite 106
    St Paul, MN 55114 1149
    USA
    +651 644 3036
    www.nacac.org

One to One
    2801 M Street NW
    Washington, DC 20007

USA
+202 338 3844
www.mentoring.org

(Information for adults interested in being mentors – mentoring a child means being involved in their life, for example befriending or tutoring, but not to the same extent as fostering or adopting)

Big Brothers/Big Sisters of America (mentoring)
    230 North 13th Street
    Philadelphia, PA 19107
    USA
    +215 567 7000
    www.bbbsa.org

Biological Clock Anxiety

Single Mothers by Choice or Chance
    PO Box 1642
    Gracie Square Station
    New York, NY 10028
    USA
    +212 988 0993
    www.singlemothers.org

Resolve
  1310 Broadway
  Somerville, MA 02144-1731
  USA
  +617 623 0744
  www.resolve.org

*American Association of Marriage
and Family Therapists*
  1133 15th Street NW
  Suite 300
  Washington, DC 20005
  USA
  +800 374 2638
  www.aamft.org

Concerned Counseling
  +888 415 8255
  http://concernedcounseling.
  com

Complementary Therapies

*National Clearing House for
Complementary and Alternative
Medicine*
  PO Box 8218
  Silver Spring MD 20907-
  8218
  USA
  +888 664 6226

www.nccam.nih.gov

*Harvard University's Mind/body
Center for Women's Health*
  The Mind/Body Program for
  Infertility
  +617 632 9530/9543
  www.mindbody.harvard.edu

Whole Person Fertility Program
  Niravi Payne
  100 Remson Street
  Brooklyn, NY 11201
  USA
  +800 666 HEALTH
  Phone consultations +941
  472 7792
  www.niravi.com

Joan Borysenko PhD
  Mind-Body Health Sciences,
  Inc
  393 Dixon Road
  Boulder, CO 80302
  USA
  +303 440 8460
  www.joanborysenko.com

Diabetes

National Diabetes Information Clearing House (NDIC)
    1 Information Way
    Bethesada, MD 20892-3560
    USA
    +301 654 3810
    www.diabetes.org

Diabetes links
    www.mendosa.com/org.htm

Eating Disorders

    National Eating Disorders
    Association
    603 Stewart St, Suite 803
    Seattle, WA 98101
    +206 382 3587
    www.nationaleatingdisorders.
    org

Eating Disorder Recovery
    +888 520 1700
    www.edrecovery.com

Fertility and Preconceptual Care

The Fertility Institute
    6020 Bullard Avenue
    New Orleans, LA 70128
    USA
    +800 375 0048
    www.fertilityinstitute.com

American Fertility Society (AFS)
    2140 11 Avenue South
    Suite 200
    Birmingham, AL 53205-2800
    USA
    +205 933 8484

Fertility information and support websites:
    www.preconception.com
    www.obgyn.net

Infertility

American Infertility Association
    666 Fifth Avenue, Suite 278
    New York, NY 10103
    USA
    +718 621 5083
    www.americaninfertility.org

American Society for Reproductive Medicine
    409 12th Street SW, Suite 203
    Washington, DC 20024-2125
    USA

+202 863 2439

www.asrm.org

Offers listings of infertility support groups, surrogacy and egg donor programs and reproductive specialists by state, plus other information.

National Infertility Network Exchange
 PO Box 204
 East Meadow, NY 11554
 USA
 +516 794 9772
 www.nine-infertility.org

International Council of Infertility Information Dissemination
 PO Box 91363
 Tucson, AZ 91363
 USA
 +520 544 9548
 www.inciid.org

Resolve
 The National Infertility Association
 1310 Broadway Avenue
 Somerville, MA 02144
 USA

+617 623 0744

www.resolve.org

The Child-Free Network
 6966 Sunrise Blvd, Suite 111
 Citrus Heights, CA 95610
 USA

Miscarriage

A.M.E.N.D.
 4324 Berrywick Terrace
 St Louis, MO 63128
 USA
 +314 487 7528

SHARE
 Pregnancy and Infant Loss Support Group
 St Joseph's Health Center
 300 First Capital Drive
 St Charles, MO 63301
 USA
 +314 947 6164
 www.nationalshareoffice.com

Support group listings
 www.kumc.edu/gec/support/miscarri.htmi

Nutrition

American Academy of Nutrition
    College of Nutrition
    3408 Sausalito
    Corona del Mar, CA 92625-
    1638
    USA
    +949 760 6788
    www.nutritioneducation.com

*Food and Nutrition Information
Center*
    National Agriculture Library
    10301 Baltimore Avenue,
    Room 30
    Beltsvile, MD 20705 2351
    USA
    +301 504 5719
    www.nal.usda.gov

Women's Health

*National Women's Health Resource
Center*
    120 Albany Street
    Suite 820
    New Brunswick, NJ 08901
    USA
    +877 986 9742
    www.healthywoman.org

Christiane Northrup, MD
Health Wisdom for Women
Philips Publishing, Inc
PO Box 60042
+7811 Montrose Road
Potomac, MD 20859-0042
USA
+800 221 8561

AUSTRALIA

PCOS

*POSAA – Polycystic Ovary Syndrome
Association of Australia*
    PO Box E140
    Emerton NSW 2770
    Australia
    +61 2 4733 4342
    www.posaa.asn.au

Adoption

*Adoption and Permanent Care
Service*
    Department of Community
    Services
    Level 9, Signature Tower
    2–10 Wentworth Street
    Parramatta NSW 2150
    Australia

+61 2 8855 4900
www.community.nsw.gov.au/
adoptions/

Alternative Therapies

*Australasian Integrative Medicine
Association*
  Locked Bag 29
  Clayton VIC 3168
  Australia
  +61 3 9594 7561
  www.aima.net.au

Nutrition

*Australasian College of Nutritional
and Environmental Medicine*
  13 Hilton Street
  Beaumaris VIC 3193
  Australia
  +61 3 9589 6088
  www.acnem.org

Fertility

Fertility Society of Australia
  Waldron Smith Management
  61 Danks Street
  Port Melborune VIC 3207
  Australia
  +61 3 9645 6359

www.fsa.au.com

Maternity Coalition
  PO Box 1190
  Blackburn North VIC 3130
  Australia
  www.maternitycoalition.org.
  au

Infertility

*ACCESS: Australia's National
Infertility Network*
  PO Box 959
  Parramatta NSW 2124
  Australia
  +61 2 9670 2380
  www.access.org.au

Suggested Reading

Before You Conceive: The complete prepregnancy guide, John R Sussmann MD (Bantam Books)
An authoritative and comprehensive guide to boosting your fertility and reducing the risks to your baby before you get pregnant.

Bottle-feeding Without Guilt, Peggy Robin (Prima)
An uplifting and absorbing, informative read for women who can't or don't want to breastfeed.

Getting Pregnant: what you need to know right now, Neils Lauerson. MD and PhD (Fireside)
Not only addresses the needs of those who are having problems conceiving, but serves as a guide for anyone planning to have a baby now or in the future.

Help Yourself Cope with Your Biological Clock: how to make the right decision about motherhood, Theresa Cheung (Hodder and Stoughton)
How to cope positively with biological clock anxiety.

In Pursuit of Fertility: a fertility expert tells you how to get pregnant, Robert Franklin MD and Dorothy Kay Brockman (Henry Holt).
Dr Franklin, clinical professor of obstetrics and gynecology at Baylor

College of Medicine in Houston, Texas, discusses all the latest medical breakthroughs for treating infertility.

The Infertility Companion: a user's guide to tests, technology and therapies, **Anna Furse (Thorsons)**
Excellent resource for women and couples living in the UK.

Infertility: the last secret, **Anna McGrail (Bloomsbury)**
Coping with the pain and frustration when you want to have a baby and it just doesn't happen.

Natural Solutions to Infertility: how to increase your chances of conceiving and preventing miscarriage, **Marilyn Glenville, PhD (Piatkus)**
Boosting your fertility through diet and lifestyle changes.

The PCOS Diet Book: how you can use the nutritional approach to deal with polycystic ovary syndrome, **Colette Harris and Theresa Cheung (Thorsons)**
Written by women with PCOS for women with PCOS, this book shows you how to beat the symptoms of PCOS through diet and lifestyle changes.

PCOS: The hidden epidemic, **Samuel S Thatcher, MD (Perspective Press)**
Dr Thatcher is a renowned expert in reproductive endocrinology and this lengthy book, published in 2000, provides a comprehensive overview of PCOS research.

PCOS: A Woman's Guide to Dealing with Polycystic Ovary Syndrome, **Colette Harris, Dr Adam Carey (Thorsons)**
The first book to discuss PCOS and offer an effective 4-point plan to relieve symptoms and improve self-esteem.

Planning for a Healthy Baby, Belinda Barnes and Suzanne Gail Bradley (Vermillion, in association with Foresight promotion of preconceptual care)
Essential preparation for pregnancy.

The Pregnant Woman's Comfort Book, Jennifer Louden (HarperSan Francisco)
A self-nurturing guide to your emotional wellbeing during pregnancy.

Single Mothers by Choice, Jane Mattes (Times Books)
A guide book for single women who are considering, or who have chosen motherhood.

Stay Fertile Longer, Mary Kittel (Pan Macmillan)
Planning now for your pregnancy when you are ready – in your 20s, 30s, 40s or today.

6 Steps to Increased Fertility, Robert L Barbieri, MD, Alice D Domar, PhD and Kevin R Loughlin, MD (Simon and Schuster)
An especially useful book from the Harvard Medical School. The step-by-step programme uses the best in mind-body medicine to maximize your fertility.

Taking Charge of Your Fertility: the definitive guide to natural birth control and pregnancy achievement (Harper Perennial)
All the information you need to monitor your menstrual cycle – whether to achieve pregnancy, avoid pregnancy or just to get better control of your moods, your health and your life.

Wanting Another Child: coping with secondary infertility, Harriet Fishman Simons (Jossey-Blass)
A compassionate resource for couples struggling with secondary infertility.

Weight Management and Fitness Through Childbirth, Theresa Cheung (Hodder and Stoughton)
Everything you need to know about pregnancy weight management and fitness: before, during and after.

What to Expect When You're Expecting, Eilen Eisenberg, Heidi Murkoff (Workman)
The pregnant woman's bible.

The Whole Person Fertility Program: a revolutionary mind-body process to help you conceive, Niravi B Payne, MS and Brenda Lane Richardson (Three Rivers Press)
A mind-body programme based on the latest scientific research that helps women and couples discover and work through the emotional barriers to conception.

Women and Self-Esteem: understanding and improving the way we think and feel about ourselves, Linda Sanford (Viking Press).

Women's Bodies, Women's Wisdom, Christiane Northrup MD (Bantam)
A popular holistic health guide that empowers women to take control of their physical and emotional health.

Glossary

Abortion: Pregnancy loss. Spontaneous abortion is another name for miscarriage, when the loss has occurred naturally. Selective abortion is when the pregnancy, or one or more babies in a multiple pregnancy, is terminated medically.

Acne: Inflammatory condition that affects the sebaceous gland of the skin.

Adrenal gland: Gland that releases DHEA (dehydroepiandrosterone) hormone and other androgens, as well as the stress hormones cortisol and adrenaline.

Alopecia: Hair loss.

Amenorrhoea: Absence of menstrual periods.

Amino acids: Building blocks found in proteins that help build, repair and maintain tissue.

Androgens: Male hormones, such as testosterone, DHEA and androstendione, responsible for male characteristics, including hair growth, voice change and muscle development. They are found in both men and women.

Anorexia nervosa: A serious eating dysfunction whereby a person starves him or herself.

Anovulation: Lack of ovulation or monthly release of an egg from th ovary.

Antiandrogen: Blocks the effects of androgens by blocking the receptor sites or by inhibiting the production of androgens.

Artificial insemination (Alh): Artificial insemination using the husband's or partner's sperm and introducing it to the cervix by means of a syringe.

Assisted reproduction (or assisted conception): Collective term for infertility treatments.

Assisted reproduction technology: Term referring to new medical technologies (including drugs, surgery, micromanipulation, etc.).

Basal body temperature (BBT): Temperature of the body at rest.

Blood sugar: Level of glucose present in the bloodstream, used by brain and muscles as energy.

Bulimia: A serious eating dysfunction characterized by bingeing, then purging and vomiting.

Caesarean section (C-section): Named after Julius Caesar who was born this way, the term refers to surgical delivery of a baby via an incision in the lower abdominal wall, with the mother under local or general anaesthetic.

Cancer: Malignant growth of cells.

Candida albicans: A yeast-like fungus, which can be found in the vagina, causing vaginal itching, dryness and discharge, and dryness in the penis. It can also be found in the mouth and the gut.

Carbohydrates: Basic component in food, composed of chains of sugar. Short chains are referred to as simple carbohydrates and include table sugar, honey and fruit sugars. These simple sugars are converted by the body into glucose, which affects insulin levels. Long chains are called complex carbohydrates and include those found in starchy foods such as breads, cereals, potatoes, fruits and vegetables. They are broken down by the body into glucose more slowly than simple sugars, and are either used as immediate energy or stored by the body for later use.

Cervical mucus: Lubricant secreted by the cervix and vaginal walls. Cervical mucus usually changes consistency around ovulation to encourage fertilization.

Cervix: Lowermost part of uterus.

Cholesterol: Waxy substance found in animal fat. In excess it can contribute to the narrowing of the artery walls, reducing blood flow.

Clomifene citrate: An ovulation-inducing drug. Popular brand name Clomid.

Conception: The fertilization of an egg by a single sperm.

Congenital: A condition present from birth.

Contraception: The prevention of conception with drugs, barrier methods, intrauterine devices (IUDs) or natural methods (herbs, timed intercourse, etc.)

Corpus luteum: The empty follicle that once held the egg before ovulation. Responsible for secreting oestrogen and progesterone. If fertilization occurs the corpus luteum sustains the pregnancy until the placenta is formed and takes over.

Cysts: Masses in ovaries that are often filled with fluid and are often benign. Can also be found in breasts and elsewhere.

Diabetes: A condition in which the body either does not use insulin efficiently or does not produce insulin at all, resulting in abnormal blood sugar levels.

Dilation and curettage (D&C): Dilating the cervix and scraping out the lining of the uterus.

Dysmenorrhoea: Painful periods.

Ectopic pregnancy: A pregnancy occurring outside the womb. The fertilized ovum attaches itself most commonly in the fallopian tube, but may sometimes stray into the abdominal cavity.

Egg: Female sex cell, also called ovum, gamete and oocyte.

Endocrinologist: A specialist of the endocrine system, the body system that controls all hormonal secretion and function.

Endometrium: The lining of the uterus.

Enzymes: Complex proteins found in the bloodstream and tissue.

Fallopian tubes: The part of the woman's reproductive system where the egg travels to meet the sperm, be fertilized and proceed to the uterus.

Fertilization: Joining of the sperm and egg, the first step in forming an embryo.

Follicle: The sac in the ovary that contains an egg (there are hundreds).

FSH: Follicle-stimulating hormone, the hormone that tells the ovary follicle to release an egg each month. (Also the generic name for an ovulation-inducing drug, Gonal F.)

Gamete: A sperm or egg.

Gamete intrafallopian transfer (GIFT): Surgical procedure by which sperm and egg are injected directly into a woman's fallopian tubes.

Glucose: Food is digested and converted to glucose; also called blood sugar and is a source of energy.

Glycaemic index: The measure of how a standard number of calories from a food impacts on blood sugar when eaten. The faster a food is digested and the more calories it contains, the more the blood sugar level will spike.

Gonadotrophin: Substance that has a stimulating effect on the ovaries or testes.

Gonadotrophin-releasing hormone (GnRH): Substance released from the hypothalamus, the part of the brain that controls reproduction, to stimulate the pituitary to produce gonadotrophins, which in turn stimulate the ovary to produce sex steroids.

Gonal F: An ovulation-inducing drug – generic name FSH.

HCG: Ovulation-inducing drugs, Pregnyl and Profasi.

High blood pressure: A condition in which the heart pumps blood through the circulatory system at a pressure greater than normal. Normal blood pressure is usually below 140/90 mm/Hg. Also called hypertension.

Hirsutism: Excess male-type hair growth in women.

Hormone: A chemical substance produced in one organ and carried in the blood to another organ, where it exerts its effect. An example is FSH which is produced in the pituitary gland and travels via the blood to the ovary, where it stimulates the growth and maturation of follicles.

Human chorionic gonadotrophin (hCG): Substance derived from the urine of pregnant women. This is what home pregnancy tests detect to confirm pregnancy. Stimulates the corpus luteum of pregnancy to make progesterone.

Human menopausal gonadotrophin (hMG): An extract from the urine of menopausal women that contains LH and FSH. Used to stimulate ovulation.

Hyperinsulinaemia: Elevated insulin levels.

Hyperthyroidism: Condition characterized by an overactive thyroid gland.

Hypoglycaemia: Low levels of blood sugar.

Hypothalamus: A major control centre of the brain that regulates the endocrine and nervous system. Responsible for maintaining body temperature, sleep, hunger and reproduction.

In vitro fertilization (IVF): A process by which an egg is fertilized in the laboratory and then inserted back into the womb.

Insulin: A hormone secreted by the pancreas that controls blood sugar levels. Insulin converts glucose from the bloodstream into glycogen, which is stored in muscle tissue and the liver.

Insulin resistance: Failure of the body to respond properly to the insulin produced by the pancreas. Related to diabetes.

Insulin sensitizers: Group of medications originally used to treat diabetes, but now sometimes used to alleviate many PCOS-related symptoms by helping to correct insulin resistance.

Intrauterine insemination (IUI): Unfrozen, fresh sperm from partner or donor is washed and introduced into the womb via a catheter.

Laparoscopy: Surgical method involving the use of a tube with a camera on the end, known as a laparoscope.

LH: Luteinizing hormone, which is released by the pituitary gland and causes ovulation.

Menopause: When menstruation has stopped for at least one year, usually around age 45 to 50.

Menses: Monthly discharge of the unfertilized egg and the uterine lining as blood flows through the vagina.

Menstruation: Monthly cycle of hormone production and ovarian activity that prepares the body for pregnancy. If pregnancy does not occur, the uterine lining is shed, causing menses.

Metformin: An insulin-sensitizing drug known as glucophage, that allows the insulin in your body to work more effectively.

Obesity: Abnormal excess of fat, usually defined as more than 20 percent over ideal weight.

Oestradiol: A naturally occurring oestrogen, a female hormone.

Oestrogen: Female sex hormone produced by the ovary and adrenal gland that causes the development of female characteristics and also plays a role in menstruation and pregnancy.

Oligomenorrhoea: Irregular periods.

Oligozoospermia: Poor sperm count, such as 20 million per ml.

Ovarian hyperstimulation: Rare complication that develops when the ovaries are overstimulated during the use of fertility medications such as Clomid or hMG. The ovaries enlarge and produce more follicles. This causes a build up of fluid in the body, resulting in sudden weight gain, pain in the abdomen and nausea.

Ovaries: The organs of the female reproductive system that store and release eggs.

Ovulation: The release of an egg from the ovary.

Pancreas: The gland that releases insulin.

Pergonal: An ovulation-inducing drug (generic name is menotropins), containing 50 percent FSH and 50 percent LH, to stimulate the ovary to produce eggs. Used in IVF treatment.

Perimenopause: The period of months or years preceding the menopause during which time there may be emotional and physical changes, including irregular cycles and fluctuating hormone levels.

Pituitary gland: The gland in the brain that is responsible for regulating hormones associated with milk production and the menstrual cycle.

Placenta: Organ that develops within the uterus during pregnancy. It provides the fetus with nourishment, permits the elimination of waste and produces hormones needed to sustain the pregnancy.

Post-coital test: A test performed on the sperm and cervical mucus after intercourse to check for mucous hostility and sperm survival.

Progesterone: A hormone produced by the corpus luteum in the ovary, the adrenal gland and the placenta (in pregnant women). It prepares the uterus for pregnancy and sustains the pregnancy.

Progestin: Name used for certain synthetic or natural progesterone agents. Often contained in birth control pills.

Prolactin: Hormone responsible for milk production.

Prostaglandins: Chemicals that signal the uterine lining to begin shedding.

Protein: Compounds that contain amino acids. Found in all living matter, proteins are essential for growth and repair of tissue.

Provera: A synthetic progesterone used to treat progesterone deficiency, in order to thicken the lining of the uterus and promote shedding of the endometrium. (Generic name is medtroxyprogesterone)

Secondary infertility: Cases of infertility when a pregnancy has previously occurred and a child or children has/have been born.

SHGB: Sex hormone-binding globulin.

Sperm count: A measure of a man's fertility, which calculates the total number of sperm per ejaculate, as well as that percentage of sperm that are both forwardly moving (motility) and of normal shape and size (morphology).

Stein–Leventhal syndrome: The original name for PCOS, after the two doctors who first diagnosed it.

Subfertility: A state of less than normal fertility.

Testosterone: Male sex hormone responsible for the development of male characteristics.

Test-tube baby: Popular term for a baby fertilized in vitro.

Ultrasound scan: A diagnostic device that uses sound waves rather than x-rays to visualize the body. Can be done on the abdomen or vaginally.

Unexplained infertility: Cases where no pathology is found in either partner yet pregnancy isn't occurring.

Uterus: The organ of the female reproductive system where the fetus develops.

ZIFT: Zygote intrafallopian transfer. A procedure in which a woman's egg is fertilized by her partner's sperm in a petri dish. The resulting zygote is then placed back in her fallopian tube.

Zygote: The fertilized ovum, a single fertilized cell resulting from fusion of the sperm and the egg. After further division the zygote is known as an embryo.

References

1. Trent ME *et al.* Fertility concerns and sexual behavior in adolescent girls with polycystic ovary syndrome: implications for quality of life. *J Pediatr Adolesc Gynecol* 2003; **16**: 33–7.

2. Thatcher S. *PCOS: The Hidden Epidemic.* Indianapolis: Perspective Press, 2000; p.222.

3. Homburg R *et al.* The management of infertility associated with polycystic ovary syndrome. *Reprod Biol Endocrinol* 2003; **14.**

4. Polson DW *et al.* Polycystic ovaries – a common finding in normal women. *Lancet* 1988; **1**: 870–2.

5. Adams J *et al.* Prevalence of polycystic ovaries in women with anovulation and idiopathic hirsuitism. *BMJ* 1986; **293**: 355–9.

6. Wise LA *et al.* Overweight and obesity in mothers and risk of preterm birth and low birth weight infants: systematic review and meta-analyses. *BMJ* 2010; **341**: c3428

7. Czeizel AE *et al.* The effect of preconceptional multivitamin supplementation on fertility. *Int J Vitam Nutr Res* 1996; **66**: 55–8.

8. Barnea ER *et al.* Stress-related reproductive failure. *In Vitro Fertil Embryo Transf* 1991; **8**: 15–23.

9. Swan SH *et al.* The question of declining sperm density revisited: an analysis of 101 studies published 1934–1996. *Environ Health Perspect* 2000; **108**: 961–6.

10. Franks S *et al.* The genetic basis of polycystic ovary syndrome. *Hum Reprod* 1997; **12**: 2641–8.

11. Marshall K *et al.* Polycystic Ovary Syndrome: clinical considerations. *Altern MedRev* 2001; **6**: 272–92.

12. Richardson MR *et al.* Current perspectives in polycystic ovary syndrome. *Am Fam Physician* 2003; **68**: 697–704.

13. Clark A *et al.* Weight loss results in significant improvements in pregnancy and ovulation rates in anovulatory obese women. *Hum Reprod* 1995; **10**: 2705–12.

14. Kiddy DS *et al.* Improvement in endocrine and ovarian function during dietary treatment of obese women with PCOS. *Clin Endocrinol* 1992; **36**:105–11.

15.   Cikot R et al. Dutch GPs acknowledge the need for preconceptual health care. Br J Gen Pract 1999; **49**: 314.

16.   Ontario Early Child Development Research Center. Preconception and Health: Research and strategies: Best Start brochure, 2001.

17.   Oliva A et al. Contribution of environmental factors to the risk of male infertility. Hum Reprod 2001; **16**: 1768–76.

18.   Sharpe RM et al. Environment, lifestyle and infertility – an intergenerational issue. Nat Cell Biol 2002; **4**: s33–40.

19.   Bolumar F et al. Body mass index and delayed conception: a European Multicenter Study on Infertility and Subfecundity. Am J Epidemiol 2000; **151**:1072–9.

20.   Pasquali R et al. Obesity and reproductive disorders in women. Hum Reprod Update 2003; **9**: 359–72.

21.   Hartz A et al. The association of obesity with infertility and related menstrual abnormalities in women. Int J Obesity 1979; **3**: 57–73.

22.   Alieva EA et al. The effect of a decrease in body weight in patients with the polycystic ovary syndrome. Akush Ginekol (Mosk) 1993; **3**: 33–6.

23.   Foreyt J, Poston WS. Obesity, a never-ending cycle. Int J of Fertil Women's Med 1998; **48**: 111–16.

24.   Clark AM et al. Weight loss results in significant improvements in pregnancy and ovulatory rates in annovulatory obese women. Hum Reprod 1995; **10**.

25.   Clark AM et al. Weight loss in obese, infertile women results in improvements in reproductive outcome for all forms of fertility treatment. Hum Reprod 1998; **6**: 1502–5.

26.   Crosignani PG et al. Overweight and obese anovulatory women with polycystic ovaries: parallel improvements and fertility rate induced by diet. Hum Reprod 2003; **18**:1928–32.

27.   Pasquali R et al. Obesity and reproductive disorders in women. Hum Reprod Update 2003; **9**:359–72.

28.   Kiddy DS et al. Differences in clinical and endocrine features between obese and non-obese subjects with polycystic ovary syndrome: an anlaysis of 263 cases. Clin Endocrinol 1989; **32**: 213–20.

29.   Robinson S et al. Postprandial thermogenesis is reduced in polycystic ovary syndrome and is associated with increased insulin resistance. J Clin Endocrinol 1992; **36**: 537–43.

30.   Baillargeon JP et al. Obese Women With Polycystic Ovary Syndrome Can Lose Weight With A Doctor's Help. The Endocrine Society, 2009.

31.   Davy B et al. Clinical trial confirms effectiveness of simple appetite control method. American Chemical Society, 2010.

32.   Bray G et al. Obesity and reproduction. Hum Reprod 1997; **12**: 26–32.

References

33. Bredella MA et al. Belly fat puts women at risk for osteoporosis, study finds. . Radiological Society of North America, 2010. *ScienceDaily*

34. Powell L et al. Lifestyle Factors and 5-Year Abdominal Fat Accumulation in a Minority Cohort: The IRAS Family Study. *Obesity*, 2011; DOI: 10.1038/oby.2011.171

35. Seymour EM et al. Blueberries May Help Reduce Belly Fat, Diabetes Risk. University of Michigan, 2009. *ScienceDaily.*

36. Hunter, G et al. Exercise training prevents regain of visceral fat for 1-year following weight loss. *Obesity.* 2010. **18 (4)**: 690–5.

37. Moran LJ et al. The obese patient with infertility: a practical approach to diagnosis and treatment. *Nutr Clin Care* 2002; **5**: 290–7.

38. Warren MP et al. The effects of intense exercise on the female reproductive system. *J Endocrinol* 2001; **170**: 3–11.

39. Holmes T et al. Relations of exercise to body image and sexual desirability among a sample of university students. *Psychol Rep* 1994; **74**: 920–2.

40. Tyrer LB et al. Nutrition and the pill. *J Reprod Med* 1984; **29**: 547–50.

41. British Medical Association. *Concise Guide to Medicines and Drugs.* London: Dorling Kindersley, 1998: p.147.

42. Sozen I et al. Hyperinsulinism and its interaction with hyperandrogenism in polycystic ovary syndrome. *Obstet Gynecol Survey* 2000; **55**: 321–8.

43. Branigan EF et al. A randomized clinical trial of treatment of clomiphene citrate-resistant anovulation with the use of oral contraceptive pill suppression and repeat clomiphene citrate treatment. *Am J Obstet Gynecol* 2003; **188**: 1424–8.

44. Latest NHS Advice available at www.nhs.uk/chq/Pages/832.aspx?CategoryID=54&SubCategoryID=127.

45. Spria N. Fertility of couples following cessation of contraception. *J Biosoc Sci* 1985; **17**: 281–90.

46. Weisberg E et al. Fertility after discontinuation of oral contraceptives. *Clin Reprod Fertil* 1982; **1**: 261–72.

47. Chasan-Tabar L et al. Oral contraceptives and ovulatory causes of delayed fertility. *Am J Epidemiol* 1997; **146**: 258–65.

48. University of Southern California School of Medicine research study. Mini pill increases risk of diabetes. *J Am Med Assoc*; 1998.

49. Barnea ER et al. Stress-related reproductive failure. *J IVF Embryo Transfer* 1991; **8**: 15–23.

50. Buck L et al. Stress reduces conception probabilities across the fertile window: evidence in support of relaxation. *Fertility and Sterility,* 2011; **95 (7)**: 2184–9

51. Jakobovits AA et al. Interactions of stress and reproduction. Zentralbl Gynakol. 2002; **124**: 189–93.

52. Lenzi A et al. Stress, sexual dysfunctions, and male infertility. J Endocrinol Invest 2003; **26**: 72–6.

53. Domar ADR et al. Distress and conception in infertile women: A complementary approach. J Am Med Wom Assoc 1999; **45**.

54. Reiko K et al. Work-related reproductive disorders among working women. Ind Health 2002; **40**: 101–12.

55. Spiegel K et al. Impact of sleep on metabolic and endocrine function. Lancet 1999; **354**: 1435–9.

56. Donga E et al A single night of partial sleep deprivation induces insulin resistance in multiple metabolic pathways in healthy subjects. Journal of Clinical Endocrinology & Metabolism, 2010; **95 (6)**: 2963–8

57. Gangwisch JE, Columbia University in New York. Sleep duration as a risk factor for diabetes incidence in a large U.S. sample. Sleep, December 2007.

58. Nakamura et al. Stress Repression in Restrained Rats by (R)-(-)-Linalool Inhalation and Gene Expression Profiling of Their Whole Blood Cells. Journal of Agricultural and Food Chemistry, 2009; **57 (12)**

59. Streeter et al. Effects of Yoga Versus Walking on Mood, Anxiety, and Brain GABA Levels: A Randomized Controlled MRS Study. The Journal of Alternative and Complementary Medicine, 2010; **16 (11)**: 1145–52.

60. For more information, please visit www.the-gi-diet.org/lowgifoods.

61. Rice R et al. Fish and a healthy pregnancy: more than just a red herring. Prof Care Mother Baby 1996; **6**: 171–3.

62. Reece MS et al. Maternal and paternal fatty acids: Possible role in pre-term birth. Am J Obstet Gynecol 1997; **176**: 907.

63. Bayer R et al. Treatment of infertility with vitamin E. Int J Fertil Womens Med 1960; **5**: 70–8.

64. Bates CJ et al. Plasma carotenoid and vitamin E concentrations in women living in a rural west African (Gambian) community. Int J of Vitam Nutr Res 2002; **72**: 133–41.

65. Rushton DH et al. Ferritin and fertility. Lancet 1991; **337**: 1554.

66. Rushton DH. Ferritin and fertility [letter]. Lancet 1991; **337**: 1554.

67. Zdziennicki A et al. Iron deficiency as a risk factor during the perinatal period. Ginekol Pol 1996; **67**: 301–3.

68. Luck MR et al. Ascorbic acid and fertility. Biol Reprod 1995; **52**: 262–6.

69. Schwabe JWR et al. Beyond zinc fingers. Trends Biochem Sci 1991; **16**: 291–6.

References

70. Kim AM et al. Zinc availability regulates exit from meiosis in maturing mammalian oocytes. *Nature Chemical Biology*, 2010; **6**: 674–81

71. Saner G et al. Hair manganese concentrations in newborns and their mothers. *Am J Clin Nutr* 1985; **41**: 1042–4.

72. Sieve BF et al. The clinical effects of a new B-complex factor, para-aminobenzoic acid, on pigmentation and fertility. *South Med Surg* 1992; 135–9.

73. Beenet M et al. Vitamin B12 deficiency, infertility and recurrent fetal loss. *J Reprod Med* 2001; **46**: 209–12.

74. Kidd GS et al. The effects of pyridoxine on pituitary hormone secretion in amenorrhea. *J Clin Endocrinol Metab* 1982; **54**: 872–5.

75. Crha I et al. Ascorbic acid and infertility treatment. *Cent Eur J Public Health* 2003; **11**: 63–7.

76. Tarin J et al. Effects of maternal ageing and dietary antioxidant supplementation on ovulation, fertilisation and embryo development in vitro in the mouse. *Reprod Nutr Dev* 1998; **38**: 499–508.

77. Battaglia C et al. Adjuvant L-arginine treatment for in-vitro fertilization in poor responder patients. *Hum Reprod* 1999; **14**: 1690–7.

78. West KP et al. Double-blind cluster randomised trial of low-dose supplementation with vitamin A or beta-carotene on mortality related to pregnancy in Nepal. *BMJ* 1999; **318**: 570–5.

79. Rothman KJ et al. Teratogenicity of high vitamin A intake. *New Engl J Med* 1995; **333**: 1369–73.

80. Howard JM et al. Red cell magnesium and glutathione peroxidase in infertile women: Effects of oral supplementation with magnesium and selenium. *Magnes Res* 1994; **7**: 49–57.

81. Roqueta-Rivera et al. Docosahexaenoic acid supplementation fully restores fertility and spermatogenesis in male delta-6 desaturase-null mice. *The Journal of Lipid Research*, 2010; **51 (2)**

82. Greening D, obstetrician and gynaecologist with sub specialist training in reproductive endocrinology and infertility at Sydney IVF, Wollongong, Australia Presented to the European Society of Human Reproduction and Embryology (ESHRE) (2009, July 1).

83. Czeizel A E et al. The effect of preconceptional multivitamin supplementation on fertility. *Int J Vitam Nutr Res* 1996; **66**: 55–8.

84. Friends of the Earth press briefing for safer chemicals campaign: *Chemicals and Health* www.foe.co.uk/resource/briefings/chemicals_and_health.pdf

85. ASH. *Smoking and Reproduction.* Research studies factsheet, 2000.

86.   Baskari L et al. Polycyclic aromatic hydrocarbon-DNA adducts in human sperm as a marker of DNA damage and infertility. Mutat Res 2003; **535**: 155–60.

87.   Howe G et al. Effects of age, cigarette smoking, and other factors on fertility: Findings in a large prospective study. BMJ 1985; **290**: 1697–9.

88.   Weinberg CR et al. Reduced fecundability in women with prenatal exposure to cigarette smoking. Am J Epidemiol 1989; **129**: 1072–8.

89.   Soares SR et al. Cigarette smoking affects uterine receptiveness. 2007 Human Reproduction **22 (2)**: 543-547

90.   Hammadeh ME et al. Protamine contents and P1/P2 ratio in human spermatozoa from smokers and non-smokers. Human Reproduction, 2010; DOI: 10.1093/humrep/deq226

91.   Mamsen LS et al. Cigarette smoking during early pregnancy reduces the number of embryonic germ and somatic cells. Human Reproduction, 2010; DOI: 10.1093/humrep/deq215

92.   Grodstein F et al. Infertility in women and moderate alcohol use. Am J Public Health 1994; **84**: 1429–32.

93.   Hatch EE, Bracken MB. Association of delayed conception with caffeine consumption. Am J Epidemiol 1993; **138**: 1082–92.

94.   Stanton CK, Gray RH. Effects of caffeine consumption on delayed conception. Am J Epidemiol 1995; **142**: 1322–9.

95.   Williams MA et al. Coffee and delayed conception [letter]. Lancet 1990; **335**: 1603.

96.   Wilcox A et al. Caffeinated beverages and decreased fertility. Lancet 1989; **1**: 840.

97.   Dixon RE et al. Inhibitory effect of caffeine on pacemaker activity in the oviduct is mediated by cAMP-regulated conductances. Brit J Pharm **163 (4)**: 745–54

98.   Fenster L et al. A prospective study of caffeine consumption and spontaneous abortion. Am J Epidemiol 1996; **143**: 525.

99.   Rasch V et al. Cigarette, alcohol, and caffeine consumption: risk factors for spontaneous abortion. Acta Obstet Gynecol Scand 2003; **82**: 182–8.

100.   Hakim, RB et al. Alcohol and caffeine consumption and decreased fertility. Fertil Steril 1998; **70**: 632–7.

101.   Joesoef MR et al. Are caffeinated beverages risk factors for delayed conception? Lancet 1990; **335**: 136–7.

102.   Gerhard I et al. Toxic pollutants, solvents and pesticides and fertility disorders. Geburtshilfe-Frauenheilked 1993; **53**: 147–60.

103.   Baranski B. Effects of workplace on fertility and related reproductive outcome. Environ Health Perspect 1993; **101**: 81–90.

104.   Kandarakis E, A et al. Endocrine Disruptors and Polycystic Ovary Syndrome (PCOS):

References

Elevated Serum Levels of Bisphenol A in Women with PCOS. *Journal of Clinical Endocrinology & Metabolism*, 2010; DOI: 10.1210/jc.2010-1658

105. Lawson C *et al*. Gene expression in the fetal mouse ovary is altered by exposure to low doses of bisphenol A. *Biology of Reproduction* 2010; DOI: 10.1095/biolreprod.110.084814

106. Adewale HB *et al*. Neonatal bisphenol-A exposure alters rat reproductive development and ovarian morphology without impairing activation of gonadotropin releasing hormone neurons. *Biology of Reproduction*, **81 (4)**: 690–9

107. Sieli PT *et al*. Comparison of serum bisphenol A concentrations in mice exposed to bisphenol A through the diet versus oral bolus exposure. *Environ Health Perspect* **119**: 1260–5.

108. Fujimoto VY *et al*. Serum unconjugated bisphenol A concentrations in women may adversely influence oocyte quality during in vitro fertilization. *Fertility and Sterility*, 2010; DOI: 10.1016/j.fertnstert.2010.11.008

109. Li DK *et al*. Occupational exposure to bisphenol-A (BPA) and the risk of self-reported male sexual dysfunction. *Human Reproduction*, 2010; **25 (2)**: 519–27.

110. Meeker JD *et al*. Semen quality and sperm DNA damage in relation to urinary bisphenol A among men from an infertility clinic. *Reproductive Toxicology*, 2010. **30 (4)**: 532–9

111. Hass U *et al*. Combined Exposure to Anti-Androgens Exacerbates Disruption of Sexual Differentiation in the Rat. *Environmental Health Perspectives*, 2010 **115**.

112. Li DK *et al*. Urine bisphenol-A (BPA) level in relation to semen quality. *Fertility and Sterility*, 2010 **95 (2)**: 625–30

113. Sieli PT *et al*. Comparison of Serum Bisphenol A Concentrations in Mice Exposed to Bisphenol A through the Diet Versus Oral Bolus Exposure. *Environmental Health Perspectives*, 2011; **119 (9)**

115. Winder C *et al*. Lead, reproduction and development. *Neurotoxicology* 1993; **14**: 303.

116. Bogden JD *et al*. Lead poisoning – One approach to a problem that won't go away. *Environ Health Perspect* 1997; **105**: 1284–7.

117. Coste J *et al*. Lead-exposed workmen and fertility: A study of 354 subjects. *Eur J Epidemiol* 1991; **7**: 154–8.

118. Ward N *et al*. Placental element levels in relation to foetal development of obstetrically normal births: A study of 39 elements. Evidence for effects of cadmium, lead and zinc on foetal growth, smoking as a cause of cadmium. *Int J Biosoc Res* 1987; **9**: 63–81.

119. Gerhard I *et al*. Heavy metals and fertility. *J Toxicol Environ Health* 1998; **54**: 593–611.

120. Choy CM *et al*. Infertility, blood mercury concentrations and dietary seafood consumption: a case-control study. *Br J Obstet Gynaecol* 2002; **109**: 1121–5.

121. Rowland AS et al. The effect of occupational exposure to mercury vapor on the fertility of female dentists. Occup Environ Med 1994; **51**: 28–34.

122. Weber RF et al. Male fertility: Possibly affected by occupational exposure to mercury. Ned Tijdschr Tandheelkd 2000; **107**: 495–8.

123. Davies BJ et al. Mercury vapor and female reproductive toxicity. Toxicol Sci 2001; **59**: 291–6.

124. Moszczynski P et al. Mercury compounds and the immune system: a review. Int J Occup Med Environ Health 1997; **10**: 247–58.

125. Castoldi A. Neurotoxic and molecular effects of methylmercury in humans. Rev Environ Health 2003; **18**: 19–31.

126. Warfninge K et al. The effect of pregnancy outcome and fetal brain development of prenatal exposure to mercury vapor. Neurotoxicology 1994; **15**.

127. Gerhard I et al. Heavy metals and fertility. J Toxicol Environ Health 1998; **54**: 593–611.

128. Sharpe RM et al. Environment, lifestyle and infertility – an inter-generational issue. Nat Cell Biol 2002; **4**: s33–40.

129. Goldhaber MK et al. The risk of miscarriage and birth defects among women who use VDU terminals during pregnancy. Am J Ind Med 1988; **13**: 695–706.

130. McDonald AD et al. Visual display units and pregnancy: evidence from the Montreal survey. Journal of Occupational Medicine 1986; **28 (12)**: 1226–31.

131. Bramwell RS et al. Visual display units and pregnancy outcome: a prospective study. J Psychosom Obstet Gynaecol 1993; **14**: 197.

132. Barnes J (in association with FORESIGHT Association for Provision of Pre-conception Care). Planning for a Healthy Baby. London: Vermillion Books, 1990: 95.

133. Furst A et al. Can nutrition affect chemical toxicity? Int J Toxicol 2002; **21**: 419–24.

134. Frisk P et al. Selenium protection against mercury-induced apoptosis and growth inhibition in cultured K-562 cells. Biol Trace Elem Res 2003; **92**: 105–14.

135. Patrick L et al. Toxic metals and antioxidants: Part II. The role of antioxidants (and zinc) in arsenic and cadmium toxicity. Altern Med Rev 2003; **8**: 106–28.

136. Sanchez-Fructuso AL et al. Lead mobilization during calcium disodium ethylenediaminetetraacetate chelation therapy in treatment of chronic lead poisoning. Am J Kidney Dis 2002; **40**: 51–8.

137. Rabbani GH et al. Antioxidants in detoxification of arsenic-induced oxidative injury in rabbits: preliminary results. J Environ Sci Health 2003; **38**: 273–87.

138. Nazrul Islam SK et al. Serum vitamin E, C and A status of the drug addicts undergoing detoxification: Influence of drug habit, sexual practice and lifestyle factors. Eur J Clin Nutr 2001; **55**: 1022–7.

References

139. Wang W et al. Retinoic acid stimulates annexin-mediated growth plate chondrocyte mineralization. *J Cell Biol* 2002; **157**: 1061–9. 107.

140. Sohlet A et al. Blood lead levels in psychiatric outpatients reduced by zinc and vitamin C. *J Orthomolec Psych* 1977; **6**: 272–6.

141. Hemingway RG. The influences of dietary intakes and supplementation with selenium and vitamin E on reproduction diseases and reproductive efficiency in cattle and sheep. *Vet Res Commun* 2003; **27**: 159–74.

142. Volesky B et al. Bio-sorption of heavy metals. *Biotechnol Prog* 1995; **3**: 235–50.

143. Quig D et al. Cysteine metabolism and metal toxicity. *Altern Med Rev* 1998; **3**: 262–70.

144. Richmond VL. Incorporation of methysulfoneylmethande sulfur into guinea pig serum proteins. *Life Sci* 1986; **39**: 263–8.

145. Lund E et al. Non-nutritive bioactive constituents of plants: dietary sources and health benefits of glucosinolates. *Int J Vitam Nutr Res* 2003; **73**: 135-43.

146. Loftus T et al. Psychogenic factors in anovulatory women: behavioral and psychanalytic aspects of anovualtory amenorrhea. *Fertil Steril* 1962; **13**: 20.

147. Cutler WB et al. Sexual behavior frequency and biphasic ovulatory type menstrual cycles. *Physiol Behav* 1985; **34**: 805–10.

148. van Roijen JH et al. Sexual arousal and the quality of semen produced by masturbation. *Hum Reprod* 1996; **11**: 147–51.

149. Baerwald AR et al. A new model for ovarian follicular development during the human menstrual cycle. 2003; 2 **80 (1)**: 116–122

150. Reported in *Psychology Today* (Jan/Feb 1996).

151. Cutler WB et al. Sexual behavior frequency and biphasic ovulatory type menstrual cycles. *Physiol Behav* 1985; **34**: 805–10.

152. Cossom J et al. How spermatozoa come to be confined to surfaces. *Cell Motil Cytoskeleton* 2003; **54**: 56–63.

153. Corty E et al. Canadian and American Sex Therapists' Perceptions of Normal and Abnormal Ejaculatory Latencies: How Long Should Intercourse Last? *J Sex Med* 2008, **5 (5)**: 1251–6

154. Stockhorst U et al. Classical Conditioning of Insulin Effects in Healthy Humans. *Psychosomatic Medicine* 1999 **61**: 424-35

155. Richardson MR et al. Current perspectives in polycystic ovary syndrome. *Am Fam Physician* 2003; **15**: 697–704.

156. Shasha SM et al. Morbidity in the ghettos during the Holocaust. *Harefuah* 2002; **141**: 364–8, 409, 408.

157. Osteria TS *et al.* Maternal nutrition, infant health, and subsequent fertility. *Philipp J Nutr* 1982; **35**: 106–11.

158. Milsom SR *et al.* LH levels in women with polycystic ovarian syndrome: have modern assays made them irrelevant? *Br J Obstet Gynaecol* 2003; **110**: 760–4.

159. Franks S. The ubiquitous polycystic ovary. *J Endocrinol* 1991; **129**: 317–19.

160. Barbieri RL *et al.* Hyperinsulinemia and ovarian hyperandrogenism. *Endocrinol Metab Clin N Am* 1988; **17**: 685–703.

161. Richardson MR *et al.* Current perspectives in PCOS. *Am Fam Physician* 2003; **15**: 697–704.

162. Sharpe RM *et al.* Environment, lifestyle and infertility – an inter-generational issue. *Nat Cell Biol* 2002; **4**: S33–40.

163. Moran LJ *et al.* Dietary composition in restoring reproductive and metabolic physiology in overweight women with polycystic ovary syndrome. *J Clin Endocrinol Metab* 2003; **88**: 812–19.

164. Cassidy A *et al.* Biological effects of a diet of soy protein, rich in isoflavones, on the menstrual cycle of premenstrual women. *Am J Clin Nutr* 1994; **60**: 333–40.

165. Aldercreutz *et al.* Dietary phytoestrogens and cancer. *J Steroid Chem Mol Biol* 1992; **41**: 331–7.

166. Auburn KJ *et al.* Indole-3-carbinol is a negative regulator of estrogen. *J Nutr* 2003; **133**: 2470–75.

167. Bitto A *et al.* Genistein aglycone does not affect thyroid function: results from a three-year, randomized, double-blind, placebo-controlled trial. *J Clin Endocrin Metabol* 2010

168. www.drnorthrup.com/womenshealth/healthcenter/topic_details.php?topic_id=59

169. Anthony MS *et al.* Soybean isoflavones improve cardiovascular risk factors without affecting the reproductive system of peripubertal rhesus monkeys. *J Nutr.* 1996; 126 (1): 43–50.

170. Chavarro JE *et al.* Soy food and isoflavone intake in relation to semen quality parameters among men from an infertility clinic. *Human Reproduction.* 2008; 23(11): 2584–90

171. Glover A *et al.* Acute exposure of adult male rats to dietary phytoestrogens reduces fecundity and alters epididymal steroid hormone receptor expression. *J Endocrinol* 2006; **189 (3)**: 565–73

172. Fraser LR *et al.* Effects of estrogenic xenobiotics on human and mouse spermatozoa. *Human Reproduction* 2006 **21**, 1184–1193.

173. Sukanya J *et al.* Assessment of Fertility and Reproductive Toxicity in Adult Female Mice after Long-Term Exposure to Pueraria mirifica Herb. *J. Reprod. Dev.* 2007; **53**, 995–1005.

References

174. Ingram DJ et al. *J Nat Cancer Inst* 1987; **79**: 1225.

175. Philips WR et al. Effect of flaxseed ingestion on the menstrual cycle. *J Clin Endocrinol Metabol* 1993; **77**: 1215–19.

176. Kidd GS et al. The effects of pyridoxine on pituitary hormone secretion in amenorrhea-galactorrhea syndrome. *J Clin Endocrinol Metabol* 1982; **54**: 872–5.

177. American Diabetics Association. Magnesium supplementation in the treatment of diabetes. *Diab Care* 1992; **15**: 1065–7.

178. Carranza-Lira S et al. The relation of the gonadotrophin response to chlormadinone according to body weight in patients with amenorrhea due to polycystic ovarian syndrome. *Eur J Gynecol Reprod Bio* 1996; **66**: 161–4.

179. Collins et al. Announced at the 13th International Congress of Dietetics, Edinburgh, Scotland (2000).

180. Hikon H et al. Antihepatotoxic actions of flavonolignans from *Silybum marianum* fruits. *Planta Medica* 1984; **50**: 248–50.

181. Clark AM et al. Weight loss results in significant improvements in pregnancy and ovulation rates in annovulatory obese women. *Hum Reprod* 1995; 2705–12.

182. Okajima T et al. Hormonal abnormalities were improved by weight loss using very low calorie diet in a patient with polycystic ovary syndrome. *Fukuoka Igaku Zasshi* 1994; **85**: 263–6.

183. Tolino A et al. Obesity and reproduction. *Acta Eur Fertil* 1994; **25**: 119–21.

184. Barnea ER et al. Stress-related reproductive failure. *J IVF Embryo Transfer* 1991; **8**: 15–23.

185. Kaplan G. Get moving with yoga. *Diab Self Manag* 2003; **20**: 28, 31–3.

186. Health benefits of meditation. *Mayo Clin Wom Healthsource* 2003; **7**: 7.

187. Hongratanaworakit T et al. Stimulating effect of aromatherapy massage with jasmine oil. *Nat Prod Commun.* 2010; **5 (1)**:157–62.

188. Hotta M et al. Carvacrol, a component of thyme oil, activates PPAR-gamma and suppresses COX-2 expression. *Journal of Lipid Research* 2010; **51 (1)**:132–9.

189. Nakamura et al. Stress Repression in Restrained Rats by (R)-(-)-Linalool Inhalation and Gene Expression Profiling of Their Whole Blood Cells. *Journal of Agricultural and Food Chemistry*, 2009; **57 (12)**: 5480–5.

190. Hongratanaworakit T et al. Relaxing effect of ylang ylang oil on humans after transdermal absorption. *Phytother Res* 2006; **20 (9)**: 758–63.

191. Hongratanaworakit T. Relaxing effect of rose oil on humans. *Nat Prod Commun* 2009; **4 (2)**: 291–6.

192. Li DJ et al. Summary of National Academic Conference on emmeniopathy and

infertility of integrated traditional Chinese and western medicine. *Zhongguo Zhong Xi Yi Jie He Za Zhi* 2001; **21**: 238–9.

193. Marshall K *et al*. PCOS: a clinical consideration. *Altern Med Rev* 2001; **6**: 272–92.

194. Czeizel AE *et al*. The effect of preconceptional multivitamin supplementation on fertility. *Int J Vitam Nutr Res* 1996; **66**: 55–8.

195. Ge XL *et al*. Treatment of secondary amenorrhea and oligohypomenorrhea with combined traditional Chinese and Western medicine. *Zhong Xi Yi Jie He Za Zhi* 1991; **11**: 645, 661–3.

196. Cahill DJ *et al*. Multiple follicular development associated with herbal medicine. *Hum Reprod* 1994; **9**: 1469–70.

197. Propping D *et al*. Treatment of corpus luteum insufficiency. *Zeitschr* 1987; **63**: 932–3.

198. Sliutz G *et al*. Agnus castus extract inhibits prolactin secretion of rat pituitary cells. *Horm Metab Res* 1993; **25**: 253–5.

199. Jarry H *et al*. In vitro prolactin but not LH and FSH release is inhibited by compounds in extracts of *agnus castus*: direct evidence for a dopaminergic principle by the dopamine receptor assay. *Exp Clin Endocrinol* 1994; **102**: 448–54.

200. Gerhard I *et al*. Mastodynon for female infertility: Randomized, placebo-controlled, clinical double-blind study. *Forsch Komplementärmed* 1998; **5**: 272–8.

201. Campbell SM *et al*. Gynecology: select topics. *Prim Care* 2002; **29**: 297–321.

202. Chaing HS *et al*. Medicinal plants: Conception/contraception. *Adv Contracept Deliv Syst* 1994; **10**: 355–63.

203. Sakai A *et al*. Induction of ovulation by Sairei-to for PCOS patients. *Endocr J* 1999; **46**: 217–20.

204. Takahashi K *et al*. Effect of TJ-68 (shakuyaku-kanzo-to) on polycystic ovarian disease. *Int J Fertil Menopausal Stud* 1994; **39**: 69–76.

205. Pinn G *et al*. Herbal medicine in pregnancy complement. *Ther Nurs Midwifery* 2002; **8**: 77–80.

206. Ushiroyama T *et al*. Effects of Unikei-to an herbal medicine on endocrine function and ovulation in women with high basal levels of luteinizing hormone secretion. *J Reprod Med* 2001; **46**: 451–6.

207. Chen BY *et al*. Acupuncture normalises dysfunction of hypothalmic-pituitary ovarian axis. *Acupunct Electother Res* 1997; **22**: 97–108.

208. Stener-Victorin E *et al*. Effects of electro-acupuncture on anovulation in women with polycystic ovary syndrome. *Acta Obstet Gynecol Scand* 2000; **79**: 180–8.

209. Liao DL *et al*. Influence of artificial cycles induced by traditional Chinese medicine on

References

the releasing and reserving gonadotrophic hormone function of the pituitary gland in the female with secondary amenorrhea. *Zhong Xi Yi Jie He Za Zhi* 1989; **9**: 458–61.

210. Jedel E *et al.* Impact of electro-acupuncture and physical exercise on hyperandrogenism and oligo/amenorrhea in women with polycystic ovary syndrome: a randomized controlled trial. *AJP: Endocrinology and Metabolism*, 2010; **300 (1)**: 37–45.

211. Manber R. Presented February 4, 2010, Society for Maternal-Fetal Medicine (SMFM) 30th Annual Meeting: The Pregnancy Meeting: Abstract 8.

212. Bergman J *et al.* The efficacy of the complex medication Phyto-Hypophyson L in female, hormone-related sterility. A randomized, placebo-controlled clinical double-blind study. *Forsch Komplementarmed Klass Naturheilkd* 2000; **7**: 190–9.

213. Kaplan B *et al*: Homoeopathy: 2. In pregnancy and for the under-fives. *Prof Care Mother Child* 1994; **4**: 185–7.

214. Sovino H *et al.* Clomiphene citrate and ovulation induction. *Reprod Biomed Online* 2002; **4**: 303–10.

215. Sidani M *et al.* Gynecology: select topics. *Prim Care* 2002; **29**: 297–321.

216. Meirow D *et al.* Ovulation induction in polycystic ovary syndrome: a review of conservative and new treatment modalities. *Eur J Obstet Gynecol Reprod Biol* 1993; **50**:123–31.

217. Nasseri S *et al.* Clomiphene citrate in the twenty-first century. *Hum Fertil* 2001; **4**: 145–51.

218. Legro RS *et al.* Clomiphene, metformin, or both for infertility in the polycystic ovary syndrome. *N Engl J Med* 2007; **356**: 551–66

219. Mohamed AFMY *et al.* Gonadotropin-releasing hormone agonist versus HCG for oocyte triggering in antagonist assisted reproductive technology cycles. *Cochrane Database of Systematic Reviews*, 2011; DOI: 10.1002/14651858.CD008046.pub3.

220. Tann SL *et al.* In-vitro maturation of oocytes from unstimulated polycystic ovaries. *Reprod Biomed Online* 2002; **4**: 18–23.

221. Tiessier MP *et al.* Comparison of follicle steroidogenesis from normal and polycystic ovaries in women undergoing IVF: relationship between steroid concentrations, follicle size, oocyte quality and fecundability. *Hum Reprod* 2000; **15**: 2471–7.

222. Diejomaoh M *et al.* The relationship of recurrent spontaneous miscarriage with reproductive failure. *Med Princ Pract* 2003; **12**: 107–11.

223. Rai R et al. Polycystic ovaries and recurrent miscarriage – a reappraisal. *Hum Reprod* 2000; **15**: 612–15.

224. Norman RJ *et al.* Lifestyle factors in the aetiology and management of polycystic ovary syndrome. In: Kovacs G (ed.). *Polycysytic Ovary Syndrome.* Cambridge: Cambridge University Press, 2000; page 103.

225. Hamilton *et al.* Association of moderate obesity with a poor pregnancy outcome in women with polycystic ovary syndrome treated with low dose gonadotrophin. *Br J Obstet Gynaecol* 1992; **99**: 128–31.

226. Tummers P *et al.* Risk of spontaneous abortion in singleton and twin pregnancies after IVF/ICSI. *Hum Reprod* 2003; **18**: 1720–3.

227. Ventura SJ *et al.* Highlights of trends in pregnancies and pregnancy rates by outcome: estimates for the United States, 1976–96. *Nat Vital Stat Rep* 1999; **47**:1–9.

228. Gupta S *et al.* Polycystic ovarian syndrome: is community care appropriate? *Int J Clin Pract* 1999; **53**: 359–62.

229. Papp Z *et al.* The evolving role of ultrasound in obstetrics/gynecology practice. *Int J Gynaecol Obstet* 2003; **82**: 339–46.

230. Turhan NO *et al.* Assessment of glucose tolerance and pregnancy outcome of polycystic ovary patients. *Int J Gynaecol Obstet* 2003; **81**: 163–8.

231. Linne Y *et al.* Natural course of gestational diabetes mellitus: long term follow up of women in the SPAWN study. *Br J Obstet Gynaecol* 2002; **109**: 1227–31.

232. Lepercq J. The diabetic pregnant woman. *Ann Endocrinol* 2003; **64**: S7–11.

233. Kasyap P *et al.* Polycystic ovary disease and the risk of pregnancy-induced hypertension. *J Reprod Med* 2000; **45**: 991–4.

234. Krizanovska K *et al.* Obesity and reproductive disorders. *Sb Lek* 2002; **103**: 517–26.

235. Wang JX *et al.* Obesity increases the risk of spontaneous abortion during infertility treatment. *Obes Res* 2002; **10**: 551–4.

236. Sadrzadeh S *et al.* Birth-weight and age at menarche in patients with polycystic ovary syndrome or diminished ovarian reserve, in a retrospective cohort. *Hum Repro* 2003; **18**: 2225–30.

237. Laitinen J *et al.* Body size from birth to adulthood as a predictor of self-reported polycystic ovary syndrome symptoms. *Int J Obes Relat Metab Disord* 2003; **27**: 710–15.

238. Jolly MC *et al.* Risk factors for macrosomia and its clinical consequences: a study of 350,311 pregnancies. *Eur J Obstet Gynecol Reprod Biol* 2003; **111**: 9–14.

239. Aortsman J *et al.* Gestational diabetes and neonatal macrosomia in the polycystic ovary syndrome. *J Reprod Med* 1991; **36**: 659–61.

240. Godfrey KM *et al.* Fetal nutrition and adult disease. *Am J Clin Nutr* 2000; **71**: 1344–52S.

241. Groenen PM *et al.* Are myo-inositol, glucose and zinc concentrations in amniotic fluid of fetuses with spina bifida different from controls? *Early Hum Dev* 2003; **71**: 1–8.

242. Artal R, MD *et al.* Obese pregnant women should gain less weight than currently recommended, researcher suggests. Commentary published in *Obstetrics & Gynecology*, January 2010.

References

243. Mullally A *et al*. Prevalence, predictors and perinatal outcomes of peri-conceptional alcohol exposure – retrospective cohort study in an urban obstetric population in Ireland. *BMC Pregnancy and Childbirth* 2011; **11**: 27

244. Bech HM *et al*. Effect of reducing caffeine intake on birth weight and length of gestation: randomised controlled trial *BMJ* 2007; **334**:409

245. Konje JC *et al*. Maternal caffeine intake during pregnancy and risk of fetal growth restriction: a large prospective observational study *BMJ* 2008; **337**.

246. Wendler CC *et al*. Embryonic caffeine exposure induces adverse effects in adulthood. *FASEB J* 2008; **23 (4)**:1272–8

247. Larsen Meyer DE *et al*. Effect of postpartum exercise on mothers and their offspring: a review of the literature. *Obes Res* 2002; **10**: 841–53.

248. May LE *et al*. Labor of love: Physically active moms-to-be give babies a head start on heart health. *FASEB J*. 2011 **24**.

249. Connor CG *et al*. Maternal antenatal anxiety and behavioural/emotional problems in children: a test of a programming hypothesis. *J Child Psychol Psychiatry* 2003; **44**: 1025–36.

250. Yu MS *et al*. Unique perspectives of women and their partners using the Prenatal Psychosocial Profile Scale. *Journal of Advanced Nursing* 2011; **67 (8)**: 1767–78

251. Crowell DT *et al*. Weight change in the postpartum period. A review of the literature. *J Nurse Midwifery* 1995; **40**: 418–23.

252. Le Quellec A *et al*. Weight loss in the post-partum period. *Rev Med Interne* 1995; **16**: 251–3

253. Amorim Adegboye AR *et al*. Cochrane Systematic Review: Losing Weight After Pregnancy: Diet And Exercise Better Than Diet Alone. July 18, 2007.

254. Barton J *et al*. What is the best dose of nature and green exercise for improving mental health? A multi-study analysis. *Environmental Science & Technology*, 2010; **44 (10)**, 3947–55

255. Algoe SB *et al*. It's the little things: everyday gratitude as a booster shot for romantic relationships. *Personal Relationships*, 2010; **17 (2)**: 217–33

256. Mosedale L. Miscarriage: the silent loss. *Child* 1993; 85–95.

257. Stack J M *et al*. The psychodynamics of spontaneous abortion. *Am J Orthopsychiatry* 1984; **54 (1)**: 162–7

258. Stay-Pederson B *et al*. *Recurrent abortion: the role of psychotherapy in early pregnancy loss – mechanisms and treatment*. London: Res Press, 1988; pp433–40.

Endnotes

a) Groundbreaking research by the University of Surrey in the UK proves this. The research looked at 367 couples who were trying to conceive over a period of three years. The women were aged 22 to 45 and the men 25 to 59. Four out of ten had a history of infertility, and the same number had suffered repeated miscarriages. Many, especially those in the older age range, came to the preconception trial as a last resort. Over the past 25 years a British organization called Foresight has pioneered an approach to human fertility that takes into account diet, exposure to pollutants, infections and nutritional status. The couples were instructed to follow a Foresight regimen that involves detoxing, being tested for mineral and vitamin deficiencies and having these put right with supplements and by eating organic food. Any infections were treated. By the end of the trial, 90 percent of these couples had given birth to healthy babies. Even 65 percent of those who had tried IVF without success became pregnant naturally.

b) Data was drawn from a large 2002 multinational study – the European Study of Daily Fecundability. It enrolled 782 women aged between 18 and 40 from seven centres: Milan, Verona, Lugano, Dusseldorf, Paris, London and Brussels. The participants kept daily records of basal body temperature and recorded the days on which intercourse and menstrual bleeding occurred. Data on 7,288 menstrual cycles contributed to the study. Among outwardly healthy couples who failed to conceive naturally within the first year, did conceive naturally in the second year, regardless of age. Research leader Dr David Dunson recommends delaying assisted reproduction until a couple has failed to conceive naturally in 18 to 24 months, as this would avoid some of the well documented side effects associated with fertility treatments, such as miscarriage and low birth weight.

c) At the University of Arkansas, 212 college students completed a survey designed to elicit information about their exercise habits, perceived sexual desirability and body image. A number of body-image items were associated with both perceived physical attractiveness and perceived sexual desirability. Total body image was related to gender, exercise level, perceived physical attractiveness, perceived sexual desirability and perception of self as a sexual partner.

d) American Scientists working at the University of Bristol suggest that women who eat fish during pregnancy are more likely to have clever children as fish contains nutrients that may enhance early brain development. But don't go overboard with oily fish. The Food Standards Agency in the UK recommends no more than three portions a week as it is thought that fish contains high levels of toxins, such as dioxins, which could be harmful for a baby to be if consumed in large quantities.

e) The Institute of Public Health, Department of Epidemiology, University of Southern Denmark, Denmark performed a study where they looked at the association between cigarette, alcohol, and caffeine consumption and the occurrence of spontaneous abortion. The conclusions were that consumption of 5 or more units alcohol per week and 375 mg or more caffeine per day during pregnancy may increase the risk of spontaneous abortion. (See website v.rasch@dadlnet.dk for more details.)

f) *New England Journal of Medicine*: In 1999 one of the first large scale studies done found that even one day after conception the chances of getting pregnant drops dramatically. At the same time researchers from the National Institute of Environmental Health Sciences in Research Park, North Carolina, also discovered that, to ensure conception, the best time to begin making love is five days prior to ovulation as well as the day of ovulation itself.

g) In one study of female infertility, 53 patients with luteal phase defect (LPD) were treated with different Chinese medicinal herbs at different phases of their menstrual cycle. The patients were treated for three menstrual cycles and there was significant improvement in the luteal phase of endometrium, and a tendency for normalization of the wave forms and its amplitude after the treatment. The findings suggested that Chinese herbal medicines capable of replenishing the kidney could regulate the hypothalamus–pituitary–ovarian axis and thus improve the luteal function. Among the 53 cases, 22 (41.5 percent) conceived, but 68.18 percent of them required other measures to preserve the pregnancy.

h) Dubai London Clinic, UAE: The objective of this study was to assess the frequency of alternative medical usage in an antenatal population. A survey of alternative medicine usage was carried out among 305 consecutive patients over 2 months at their registration in mid-pregnancy at an Australian Antenatal Clinic. The study showed that something like 40 percent of patients used alternative medical therapy, including 12 percent herbal therapy. No specific study of pregnancy outcome was carried out, but it is of concern that some herbs taken had the potential to adversely affect pregnancy outcome. The herbal therapies commonly used in preg-nancy are reviewed with their potential complications; examples of toxicity are also discussed. It is important to obtain a herbal medicine history at any time but particularly in pregnancy. Herbs may have unrecognized effects on pregnancy or labour, have interactions with prescribed medications and have potentially serious complications for the fetus.

i)   CONCLUSIONS: Metformin therapy during pregnancy in women with PCOS was safely associated with reduction in SAB and in GD, was not teratogenic, and did not adversely affect birth weight or height; or height, weight, and motor and social development at 3 and 6 months of life.

j)   The trend for elective caesareans has been made popular by celebrities, but doctors point out that babies born by c-section are seven times more likely to suffer from breathing problems. While serious complications are rare, they can include haemorrhaging, scarring and damage to the ovaries. It's also important to point out that c-section is major surgery and you will need at least four weeks to recover compared to a matter of days for women with natural births. Breastfeeding will be harder and you will need to stay in hospital for longer. Around 60 percent of women who have a caesarean will still feel pain from the wound five months later.

ABOUT THE AUTHORS

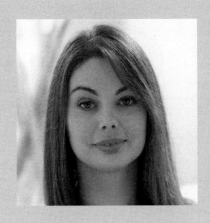 **Colette Harris** is a leading health writer and editor, who was diagnosed with PCOS in 1996, and has since then written about PCOS in international newspapers and magazines, to raise awareness of the condition. Her passion is finding practical self-help strategies based in scientific research, or expert experience, that have a profound effect on PCOS symptoms, and fertility – from nutrition to stress relief. She uses diet, exercise and herbal medicine to manage her own PCOS. She is also keen to challenge the myth that women with PCOS can't have children – as the majority can, and do, even if they need a bit of help from themselves or their healthcare professionals along the way. This book is designed to provide support along the journey. Colette is a patron of Verity, the UK charity for women with PCOS, and speaks at conferences and support groups.

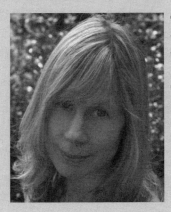 **Theresa Cheung** is a freelance writer, teacher, health consultant and mum who was diagnosed with PCOS in 1997 when she was trying to conceive. At that time, Theresa was living in the US, where she had her first child using fertility drugs. She then moved to the UK where she extended her family with the aid of continued fertility treatment.

www.verity-pcos.org.uk

JOIN THE HAY HOUSE FAMILY

As the leading self-help, mind, body and spirit publisher in the UK, we'd like to welcome you to our family so that you can enjoy all the benefits our website has to offer.

 EXTRACTS from a selection of your favourite author titles

 COMPETITIONS, PRIZES & SPECIAL OFFERS Win extracts, money off, downloads and so much more

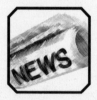 **LISTEN** to a range of radio interviews and our latest audio publications

 CELEBRATE YOUR BIRTHDAY An inspiring gift will be sent your way

 LATEST NEWS Keep up with the latest news from and about our authors

 ATTEND OUR AUTHOR EVENTS Be the first to hear about our author events

 iPHONE APPS Download your favourite app for your iPhone

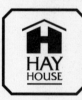 **HAY HOUSE INFORMATION** Ask us anything, all enquiries answered

join us online at **www.hayhouse.co.uk**

 292B Kensal Road, London W10 5BE
T: 020 8962 1230 E: info@hayhouse.co.uk